D0053256

ASSESSMENT OF EATING DISORDERS

ASSESSMENT *of* EATING DISORDERS

Edited by

James E. Mitchell
Carol B. Peterson

THE GUILFORD PRESS
New York London

A Division of Guilford Publications, Inc.
72 Spring Street, New York, NY 10012
www.guilford.com

Printed in the United States of America

This book is printed on acid-free paper.

Last digit is print number: 9 8 7 6 5 4 3 2 1

Library of Congress Cataloging-in-Publication Data

Assessment of eating disorders / edited by James E. Mitchell and Carol B. Peterson.
p. cm.
Includes bibliographical references and index.
ISBN 1-59385-196-0 (trade cloth)
1. Eating disorders—Diagnosis. I. Mitchell, James E. (James Edward), 1947–
II. Peterson, Carol B.
RC552.E18A83 2005
616.85′26075—dc22

2005010753

To
Darren and Amelia

About the Editors

James E. Mitchell, MD, is currently the NRI/Lee A. Christofferson MD Professor and Chair of the Department of Clinical Neuroscience at the University of North Dakota School of Medicine and Health Sciences and President and Scientific Director of the Neuropsychiatric Research Institute. Dr. Mitchell completed his undergraduate education at Indiana University and medical school at Northwestern University. Since entering academics he has focused primarily on research in the areas of eating disorders and obesity. Dr. Mitchell is on the editorial boards of the *International Journal of Eating Disorders* and the *Eating Disorders Review*. He has published more than 300 articles and book chapters and is the author or editor of nine books. Dr. Mitchell is currently funded by the National Institutes of Health for his research on bulimia nervosa, binge eating disorder, bariatric surgery, and genetic studies in individuals with eating disorders.

Carol B. Peterson, PhD, received her doctorate in clinical psychology from the University of Minnesota. She is currently a research associate in the Eating Disorders Research Program at the University of Minnesota, where her investigations have focused on the assessment, diagnosis, and treatment of bulimia nervosa, anorexia nervosa, binge eating disorder, and obesity. Dr. Peterson has authored more than 45 articles and book chapters and has served as an investigator on several federally funded research projects focusing on eating disorders. She is also an adjunct assistant professor in the Department of Psychology at the University of Minnesota and has a part-time private practice in which she specializes in the treatment of eating disorders.

Contributors

Guy Cafri, MA, Department of Psychology, University of South Florida, Tampa, Florida

Ross D. Crosby, PhD, Neuropsychiatric Research Institute, Fargo, North Dakota

Scott Crow, MD, Department of Psychiatry, University of Minnesota School of Medicine, Minneapolis, Minnesota

Jill M. Denoma, MS, Department of Psychology, Florida State University, Tallahassee, Florida

Scott G. Engel, PhD, Neuropsychiatric Research Institute, Fargo, North Dakota

Kathryn H. Gordon, MS, Department of Psychology, Florida State University, Tallahassee, Florida

Carlos M. Grilo, PhD, Department of Psychiatry, Yale University School of Medicine, New Haven, Connecticut

Thomas E. Joiner, Jr., PhD, Department of Psychology, Florida State University, Tallahassee, Florida

Daniel le Grange, PhD, Department of Psychiatry, University of Chicago, Chicago, Illinois

Leslie J. Heinberg, PhD, Department of Epidemiology and Biostatistics, Division of Public Health, Case Western Reserve University, Cleveland, Ohio

James E. Mitchell, MD, Department of Clinical Neuroscience, University of North Dakota School of Medicine and Health Sciences, Fargo, North Dakota

Carol B. Peterson, PhD, Department of Psychiatry, Eating Disorder Research Program, University of Minnesota, Minneapolis, Minnesota

Cheryl L. Rock, PhD, Department of Family and Preventive Medicine, University of California–San Diego, San Diego, California

Megan Roehrig, MA, Department of Psychology, University of South Florida, Tampa, Florida

Dana A. Satir, BA, Department of Psychiatry, College of Physicians and Surgeons, Columbia University, and Eating Disorders Research Unit, New York State Psychiatric Institute, New York, New York

Susan Swigart, MD, Department of Psychiatry, University of Minnesota School of Medicine, Minneapolis, Minnesota

J. Kevin Thompson, PhD, Department of Psychology, University of South Florida, Tampa, Florida

B. Timothy Walsh, MD, Department of Psychiatry, College of Physicians and Surgeons, Columbia University, and Eating Disorders Research Unit, New York State Psychiatric Institute, New York, New York

Stephen A. Wonderlich, PhD, University of North Dakota School of Medicine and Health Sciences and Neuropsychiatric Research Institute, Fargo, North Dakota

Preface

When we initially developed this project, it was clear to us that assessment of eating disorders is an important topic that has not been adequately addressed. Eating disorder symptoms are often quite complex and require a variety of forms of assessment, some of which are atypical for most patients with emotional problems. Therefore, we thought that a text devoted to this topic that offered a thorough discussion of various aspects of assessment as well as techniques would provide clinicians and researchers alike with a work of practical importance. While much of what is included in this text is evidence based, we have attempted to present this information in such a way that it will be helpful for researchers, students, and practicing clinicians.

The first two chapters of this book include diagnostic and classification issues. B. Timothy Walsh (Chapter 1, with Dana A. Satir) chaired the DSM-IV workgroup on eating disorders and has been a leader in the field on the topic of diagnostic issues as the criteria have evolved. Chapter 2, by Kathryn H. Gordon, Jill M. Denoma, and Thomas E. Joiner, Jr., focuses more on issues of scientific validity.

Chapter 3, by Carol B. Peterson, describes in depth the process of diagnostic interviewing. The diagnostic interview of a patient with an eating disorder requires a thorough assessment of many factors that are not typically included in a standard psychiatric interview. In Chapter 4, James E. Mitchell focuses on providing a database that can be used by clinicians as a way of obtaining additional information about patients.

Chapter 5, by Carlos M. Grilo, and Chapter 6, by Carol B. Peterson and James E. Mitchell, discuss structured, semistructured, and self-report measures. Although the use of these instruments has usually been restricted to research settings, such measures are finding their way into clinical practice with increasing frequency and are allowing clinicians to better formulate treatment plans and to evaluate outcomes, both for clinical purposes and for documentation.

Chapters 7 and 8 provide an overview of the medical evaluation of patients with eating disorders, clearly of great clinical importance, particularly in patients with anorexia nervosa, and the nutritional assessment that is essential in terms of both assessment and treatment planning. Scott Crow and Susan Swigart (Chapter 7) and Cheryl L. Rock (Chapter 8) bring backgrounds with considerable clinical and research experience in these areas.

Daniel le Grange outlines family assessment in Chapter 9. While working at the Maudsley Hospital in London, Dr. le Grange was part of the early treatment trials of the Maudsley family therapy approach and has devoted much of his career to the assessment and treatment of families. J. Kevin Thompson, who has conducted some of the most important work in the area, reviews the assessment of body image disturbance in Chapter 10 with his colleagues Megan Roehrig, Guy Cafri, and Leslie J. Heinberg. In Chapter 11, Scott G. Engel, Stephen A. Wonderlich, and Ross D. Crosby present information on the use of ecological momentary assessment, a new way of assessing patients with eating disorders that until recently has been primarily a research tool but will be finding its way into clinical settings in the next few years. Finally, in Chapter 12, James E. Mitchell integrates this information and provides strategies for treatment planning based on assessment.

We have tried to be comprehensive and scholarly but at the same time have attempted to distill what we think are the most important useful elements for clinicians. We hope you find that this text helpful in your clinical work and research with patients with eating disorders.

JAMES E. MITCHELL
CAROL B. PETERSON

Contents

ASSESSMENT OF EATING DISORDERS

CHAPTER 1

Diagnostic Issues

B. Timothy Walsh
Dana A. Satir

Patients with eating disorders may present in a variety of settings with complex histories and a range of symptoms. While the two most well-defined syndromes, anorexia nervosa (AN) and bulimia nervosa (BN), are readily recognizable if a full history is available, patients frequently do not provide a complete description of their difficulties. They may describe symptoms that suggest the presence of other diagnoses, and they may fail to meet all criteria for AN or BN. The goal of the clinical assessment is to elicit information that will permit the accurate description of presenting symptoms, the identification of specific syndromes, and appropriate treatment recommendations. This chapter reviews the evaluation and assessment of patients with disordered eating in a general clinical setting. The clinician may also wish to consider the use of structured diagnostic and assessment instruments routinely employed in research settings. These are described elsewhere in this volume.

We first provide a broad description of the clinical assessment of the symptoms and signs associated with eating disorders. We then identify specific issues particularly relevant to the different eating disorder categories as identified by DSM-IV (the fourth edition of the *Diagnostic and Statistical Manual of Mental Disorders*; American Psychiatric Association, 1994). We thereby hope to provide a useful introduction to the evaluation of patients with disordered eating.

PSYCHIATRIC INTERVIEW

The clinical assessment of individuals with eating disorders should follow the standard approach to the assessment of any emotional or behavioral problem, but the content and specific questions should be tailored to focus on eating disorders. One major goal of the initial assessment is to allow the patient to provide a description of the development of his/her difficulties from his/her perspective. Opportunities to corroborate aspects of this story can be pursued by consulting the patient's family, if possible and appropriate, the referring clinician, and previous treatment providers. A primary focus of the evaluation should be the patient's weight and eating history and associated emotional and behavioral problems.

Reason for the Assessment (Chief Complaint)

The assessment should begin by determining, from the patient's perspective, what prompted the evaluation. One of the difficult aspects in treating individuals with eating disorders, especially with AN, is patients' ambivalence about making changes in their eating, coupled with a tendency to deny the potentially serious nature of their disorder. Clarification of whether the patient initiated the appointment or was persuaded by another party to come for an evaluation can assist the clinician's assessment of the patient's insight and level of commitment to change. This discussion also provides an opportunity for the patient to express his or her feelings about the assessment. If the patient denies any understanding of the reason for an evaluation, expresses annoyance at having to speak with the clinician, or does not perceive a significant clinical problem, the assessment may be particularly challenging. In such instances, the clinician should display empathic support by assuring the patient that the clinician is not making any value judgments about the patient or the patient's behavior, and that together they can better understand why other people are concerned about the patient's health and well-being. Even if the clinician views the presenting symptoms differently from the way the patient does, as is often the case, the opportunity for an empathic dialogue may assist in the formation of an alliance.

History of the Current Illness

Once the patient's understanding of the reason for the assessment has been established, the clinician can begin to elicit the history of the development of eating symptoms. Because concerns about body image and cognitive disturbances regarding shape and weight are virtually universal among individuals with eating disorders, it is important to obtain a history of changes in weight and dieting as well as current eating patterns. This can begin with open-ended questions about changes in eating habits and weight in the recent past or during the current disordered eating episode. The clinician should also ask for descriptions of events or experiences (e.g., emotional or environmental) that the patient believes may have contributed to the development or exacerbation of the problem. As the onset of an eating disorder is frequently associated with a significant life change or interpersonal event, the clinician should ask the patient to describe what was going on at the time that symptoms began, and to consider whether personal life events may have had a direct or indirect influence on the evolution of eating symptoms.

In assessing individuals with disordered eating, it is very important to obtain a picture of the patient's current eating habits by asking the patient to describe the frequency and content of meals and snacks on a recent, typical day. The clinician should also specifically inquire about several eating-related behaviors:

1. The degree to which the individual restricts calorie intake, and whether he or she avoids specific foods and/or categories of foods. Many individuals with eating disorders avoid foods they believe to be high in calories, such as desserts and red meats. A smaller number develop vegetarianism or other restrictive eating patterns during the course of their disorder. The clinician should also inquire about religious food restrictions (e.g., keeping kosher) and reported allergies to foods.
2. The occurrence and frequency of binge eating. Although the definition of a binge in DSM-IV explicitly requires the consumption of an objectively large amount of food, many individuals refer to the consumption of a modest or even small amount of food they had not intended to eat as a binge. The clinician should ascertain what is consumed during a typical episode of binge eating.
3. The occurrence and frequency of purging behaviors, such as self-induced vomiting and laxative or diuretic abuse. The clinician may also inquire about less common methods such as the use of syrup of ipecac, which is employed by some individuals to help induce vomiting, the omission of hypoglycemic agents (e.g., insulin) by diabetics, and the practice of chewing and spitting out food without swallowing.
4. The frequency and intensity of exercise, and how exercise patterns have changed in relation to changes in eating habits and weight.

In obtaining a history of the development of eating symptoms, several other topics should at least briefly be raised as they are often of importance in the development of the disorder. These include the highest and lowest weights, at least at the current height, and (for females) the age at which menstruation started. The clinician should inquire about any sustained (longer than 3 months) episodes of amenorrhea, and the association of such episodes with weight changes. This information is important not only in establishing the onset and duration of illness but also in putting into context the patient's current presentation. Because the patient's experience of his or her shape and weight are important in both the onset and maintenance of eating-disordered thoughts and behaviors, the clinician should ask what weight the patient thinks would be ideal, and the patient's view of him- or herself at the current weight.

Two other areas warranting attention are the patient's family history of eating attitudes and behaviors and the patient's occupational and social history. Often the family's attitudes toward eating and accompanying behaviors (e.g., dieting), especially if taken to an extreme, can play a significant role in the formation of patients' attitudes and behaviors. The clinician should inquire about these family patterns, if not already volunteered by the patient, and their effect on his or her relationship to food. Similarly, the emphasis on shape and weight within the family structure and its influence on the patient's perceptions of shape and weight should be discussed.

Patients with eating disturbances frequently engage in occupations in which shape and weight are highly emphasized (e.g., personal trainer) or food is the focal point (e.g., waitress). Whether the pursuit of such careers is a contributing factor to or a by-product of the eating disturbance undoubtedly varies, but the relationship of these occupations to the chronology of changes in eating and dieting practices should be reviewed. Such information may prove valuable in treatment planning when a consideration of career plans can be more thoroughly evaluated.

Medical Complications

Eating disorders, especially AN, are associated with significant medical problems. The clinician should ask whether the patient has experienced any physical problems as a consequence of the eating disturbance, and specifically inquire about any emergency room visits or less acute medical care, and about the existence of complications such as osteoporosis and dental disease.

Treatment History

Most assessments of individuals presenting for an evaluation will uncover symptoms of a possible eating disorder. If so, the clinician should obtain information about any treatments attempted. A range of treatment settings (e.g., inpatient, day-program, outpatient), modalities (e.g., behavioral, cognitive, interpersonal, family-oriented, psychopharmacological, medical) and intensity are currently employed in the treatment of eating disorders. Often, these are difficult for the patient (or clinician) to characterize accurately. Furthermore, for a patient with a long history of illness, the complete history of treatment may be too lengthy to obtain in a single assessment. It is important to ascertain whether and how often the patient has been hospitalized for treatment of the eating disorder or its complications, what psychological strategies and medication interventions have been attempted, and what the patient has found to be most and least helpful. It is also useful to determine the reason for termination of treatment. For example, did insurance coverage expire? Did the patient leave treatment against medical advice? Such information can often be used to help judge the severity of the disorder and the patient's willingness to engage in treatment.

Coexisting Conditions

Because of the frequent occurrence of disturbances of mood and of substance abuse among individuals with eating disorders, symptoms of these disorders should be explicitly reviewed. Specific questions about the lifetime usage of alcohol and recreational drugs should be posed. The clinician should be mindful about patients' potential reluctance to disclose such information, but should inquire directly, in a nonjudgmental fashion ("Have you ever tried marijuana, cocaine, or other recreational drugs?"). The clinician should also be alert for indications of personality disorders, which are commonly present among individuals with eating disturbances.

Physical Assessments

The approach just described should provide a description, largely based on the patient's report, of the current eating difficulties and their history and development, a description of other major psychological and medical problems, and an outline of current and past treatments. An important additional component of the assessment is the acquisition of more objective measures of current health status. These include (1) height and weight, (2) vital signs (pulse, blood pressure), (3) general physical examination, and (4) laboratory tests. Some or all of these measures can be obtained by the clinician assessing the history, if he or she has the requisite training and experience, or from a physician who serves a general medical role. How imperative it is to obtain these assessments depend on the nature of the presenting problem and the clinician's observations of the patient. For example, a patient with a history of substantial weight loss or of frequent purging is in more urgent need of physical assessment than one with a normal and stable weight but psychological overconcern with shape and weight. Additional details regarding the medical complications specific to each disorder are provided later in this chapter.

Patient Reluctance to Provide Information

For a variety of reasons, patients may be reluctant to provide accurate information about their difficulties. In some instances, patients are ashamed of beliefs or behaviors that they recognize as abnormal but feel unable to control. Patients may deny that they purge or that they use recreational drugs, or they may claim to weigh more than they do do—and consume excessive amounts of liquids or carry concealed objects when they are weighed. No approach to such denial and subterfuge is universally effective. However, it may be useful for the clinician to note that individuals with eating problems commonly find it difficult to be open about all aspects of their problems, and, in a nonconfrontational manner, ask if there are issues the patient has difficulty admitting. The clinician should avoid criticizing the patient for not being open, as such maneuvers are unlikely to yield more accurate information and will undermine the development of a therapeutic alliance.

DIFFERENTIAL DIAGNOSIS

Before concluding that the patient's difficulties are best ascribed to the existence of an eating disorder, the clinician should consider two other possibilities: that the eating disturbances are better considered as symptoms of another psychiatric disorder or that the symptoms are secondary to a general medical condition. For example, episodes of overeating (binge eating episodes) may occur in association with major depressive disorder, and weight loss is a prominent symptom of a variety of medical illnesses. When a complete history is available, typical cases of AN and BN are usually easy to recognize. However, when the history is unclear or the features are unusual, the clinician should seriously consider the possibility that another diagnosis is warranted. The following sections provide some specific considerations about the differential diagnosis of AN and BN.

Anorexia Nervosa

Diagnosis

DSM-IV specifies four major criteria for the diagnosis of AN. The most prominent is a refusal to maintain a minimally acceptable body weight for a person's height and age. DSM-IV recommends a guideline of 85% of ideal body weight (IBW) but does not provide a more specific standard. The 10th edition of the *International Classification of Mental and Behavioural Disorders* (ICD-10; World Health Organization, 1992) requires that patients have a body mass index (BMI) equal to or below 17.5 kg/m^2, a criterion considerably more stringent than that of DSM-IV, especially in light of current recommendations for desirable body weight (Metropolitan Life Insurance Company, 1983). This variability, and the fact that DSM-IV explicitly describes the 85% of IBW only as an example, indicate that clinical judgment should be exercised in determining whether the patient is sufficiently underweight to meet this criterion. This is particularly true in the assessment of children and adolescents whose normal weight goal is influenced by the demands of growth and the stage of pubertal development. It is also important to consider the patient's weight history and, for females, the weight at which menses were regular in assessing the relative "normality" of the current weight.

The clinician should be aware that severe malnutrition itself is associated with profound psychological and cognitive disturbances. Underweight patients may exhibit delays in speech, illogical thought patterns, and a limited range of affect. It may be useful to draw the patient's attention to some of these consequences of maintaining an undernourished state as a way to help foster greater insight. Similarly, it may be helpful to note how the eating disturbance has interfered with other facets of the patient's life.

For the diagnosis of AN, DSM-IV requires that there be an intense fear of gaining weight. In classic cases, this fear is overt and acknowledged by the patient. However, other individuals with AN deny that they are afraid of gaining weight, and may even describe attempts to increase calorie consumption. On the other hand, focused questioning about what foods the patient actually consumes and about the patient's emotional reaction to increases in weight often suggests a deeply seated concern about weight gain. Similarly, the accounts of family members regarding the patient's attitudes and eating behavior may yield evidence of strong fears of weight gain. A patient's insistence, even in the face of persuasive accounts of behaviors that suggest the contrary, that he or she is not afraid of gaining weight may raise questions about whether this DSM-IV criterion for AN is satisfied. The clinician should exercise clinical judgment and assign the diagnosis of AN if all other criteria are met and there is substantial, even indirect, evidence of fear of gaining weight.

DSM-IV also requires evidence of what is usually described as a distortion of body image. This may be manifested in a variety of ways, including the patient's feeling that, despite being underweight, a part of the body is too fat, or by denying how serious the currently low body weight actually is. Sufficient information to assess these psychological characteristics will usually have been obtained during the discussion of the current illness described earlier.

DSM-IV requires that, for the diagnosis of AN, postmenarchal women have amenorrhea for at least 3 months, a requirement that highlights the importance of obtaining a menstrual history during the evaluation. It should be noted, however, that considerable debate continues regarding the appropriateness of this criterion in making a clinical diagnosis of AN (Garfinkel et al., 1996a; Cachelin & Maher, 1998; Watson & Andersen, 2003).

DSM-IV suggests that individuals with AN be classified into one of two mutually exclusive subtypes: the restricting subtype (AN-R) and the binge–purge subtype (AN-BP). In most eating disorders centers, one quarter to one half of patients with AN are classified as having the binge–purge subtype. Because of uncertainty about the characteristics of binge eating associated with AN, DSM-IV does not specify a frequency and duration criteria for binge-eating episodes. DSM-IV also does not indicate whether what constitutes an "unusually large amount of food" should take into account the patient's low weight. There is considerable empirical support for this subtype distinction, as individuals with the AN-BP subtype report more mood disturbances and impulsive behaviors than those with the AN-R subtype (see DaCosta & Halmi, 1992, for review). However, it is common for someone who initially presents with the AN-R subtype to develop binge eating and purging if the illness persists for several years and therefore for his or her subtype classification to change. If this behavioral change is also accompanied by an increase in weight to within a normal range, a change in the diagnosis from AN to BN may be warranted.

Physical Examination

The underweight state that is a defining characteristic of AN is associated with significant findings on physical examination. The most striking is often the obvious wasting. Blood pressure, pulse, and body temperature can be impressively low. The hair may be thin and brittle, and "lanugo"—fine, downy hair—may be present on the trunk, face, and extremities. Enlarged salivary glands may make the face appear disproportionately full in light of the degree of malnutrition. The hands and feet may be cold and blue (acrocyanosis), and there may be peripheral edema.

Laboratory Abnormalities

Virtually all the body's physiological systems are disrupted by the undernutrition of AN, and laboratory assessments of these systems will typically show abnormalities. The assessment of the patient's physical state (see Chapter 7) is an important part of the evaluation. For other reviews of this topic, see Walsh (2001) and Halsted (2001).

Differential Diagnosis

Before concluding that the symptoms of disordered eating are best ascribed to AN, the clinician should consider other Axis I psychiatric disorders and general medical conditions. Many serious medical illnesses are associated with substantial weight loss, but relatively few typically occur in adolescents and young adults. Examples of general medical conditions that should be considered include gastrointestinal illnesses such as Crohn's disease, brain tumors, malignancies, and AIDS. The intense psychological reward associated with losing weight and the fear of weight gain, which are prominent in typical AN, are not characteristic of these conditions. However, the presence of atypical psychological features should prompt a greater concern about the possibility that the weight loss is not due to AN.

Other Axis I mental disorders, such as major depressive disorder and schizophrenia, may occasionally be associated with weight loss and disturbances in eating behavior. However, these disorders are not associated with the concerns about shape and weight characteristic of AN. Some of the psychological characteristics of individuals with social phobia, obsessive–compulsive disorder (OCD), and body dysmorphic disorder (BDD) resemble those of AN. However, individuals with these disorders do not exhibit the unrelenting drive for thinness and the low body weight that are defining characteristics of AN. There is great similarity between the psychological features of AN and those of BN. However, in the DSM-IV system, a diagnosis of BN is not made in the presence of AN, which results in a distinction that is often based on body weight: below normal in AN, normal or above normal in BN.

Bulimia Nervosa

Diagnosis

The salient diagnostic feature of BN is the repeated occurrence of episodes of binge eating followed by inappropriate behavior aimed at preventing weight gain. To determine whether the patient's symptoms fulfill this criterion, it is crucial to obtain a good description of current eating behavior. DSM-IV requires that a binge comprise an amount of food "definitely larger than most people would eat during a similar period of time and under similar circumstances" (American Psychiatric Association, 1994, p. 594). Clearly, this is not a precise definition, and it requires the clinician to exercise judgment in deciding whether or not the criterion is met. The second DSM-IV requirement for a binge is that the eating during a binge must be associated with a sense of loss of control over the eating. The assessment of this feature is reasonably straightforward, as it only requires an inquiry into the patient's subjective state while binge eating. In fact, several studies (e.g., Beglin & Fairburn, 1992; Gleaves, Williamson, & Barker, 1993) have found that most individuals associate a sense of loss of control over the eating as a more important characteristic of a 'binge' than the amount of food consumed, emphasizing the need for the clinician to assess both characteristics.

The DSM-IV criteria for a binge also require that it occurs within a discrete period of time and suggest a period of less than two hours. Therefore, the consumption of a large amount of food over the course of a day achieved by continuous snacking on small amounts of food would not meet criteria for a binge-eating episode.

DSM-IV requires that the episodes of binge eating (as well as the inappropriate compensatory behaviors) must occur at a minimum average frequency of twice weekly for the 3 months prior to the evaluation. There is concern that this frequency threshold is too demanding, as data suggest that individuals who engage in binge eating and purging once a week share many clinical characteristics with those who engage in such behaviors more frequently (Crow, Agras, Halmi, Mitchell, & Kraemer, 2002).

The most common compensatory behaviors described by patients with BN presenting to eating disorder clinics are self-induced vomiting and, much less frequently, laxative abuse. Uncommonly employed methods include diuretic abuse, and, among individuals with Type I diabetes mellitus, the omission of insulin. All these examples are considered methods of purging, as they result, to a variable degree, in a loss of nutrients from the body.

Within the definition of inappropriate compensatory behavior, DSM-IV also includes nonpurging behavior such as fasting or excessive exercise. Examples might include engaging in physical activity after a binge that the patient would not ordinarily pursue or consuming no food for 24 hours following a binge. While such nonpurging behavior has been described, it is difficult to distinguish excessive from normal exercise and fasting from strict dieting. For these reasons, relatively little is known about the characteristics of nonpurging behaviors, or of individuals with BN who employ only nonpurging methods to compensate for binge eating.

On the basis of whether or not the individual employs purging methods to compensate for binge eating, DSM-IV suggests that patients with BN be classified as belonging to one of two mutually exclusive subtypes, purging or nonpurging. Patients with the purging subtype have greater levels of comorbid psychopathology and a higher risk of physical complications, such as electrolyte imbalances, than patients with the nonpurging subtype (Garfinkel et al., 1996b).

In addition to these behavioral disturbances, DSM-IV requires that individuals display an overconcern with body shape and weight, very similar to that of individuals with AN. While body image plays an important normal role in the regulation of self-esteem, individuals with BN overvalue shape and weight compared to individuals without eating disorders.

Medical Complications

Self-induced vomiting over many years may lead to softening and erosion of dental enamel, especially on the lingual surfaces of upper front teeth. In some patients, binge eating and vomiting is associated with enlargement of salivary glands. The development of calluses on the dorsum of the hand has been described among individuals who, in manually stimulating the gag reflex, rub the hand against the teeth.

Laboratory Abnormalities

Frequent purging is associated with fluid and electrolyte abnormalities, including hypokalemia, hyponatremia, and hypochloremia (American Psychiatric Association, 1994).

Differential Diagnosis

Individuals with BN share many psychological and behavioral characteristics with those who have the binge–purge subtype of AN. The major distinguishing feature is the abnormally low weight of patients with AN. However, the line between the binge–purge subtype of AN in partial remission and current BN is very unclear.

Other medical and neurological conditions such as Kleine–Levin syndrome are associated with binge eating but are not accompanied by the inappropriate compensatory behavior and the overconcern with shape and weight that characterize BN. Similarly, overeating sometimes occurs in association with major depressive disorder with atypical features and with borderline personality disorder, but is usually not associated with the other behavioral and psychological characteristics of BN. On the other hand, if criteria both for BN and for another mental disorder are met, both diagnoses should be given.

Binge Eating Disorder

While not an official DSM-IV diagnostic category, binge eating disorder (BED) has received considerable attention in recent years, prompted at least in part by the alarming rise in the prevalence of obesity. BED is characterized by recurrent binge eating episodes in the absence of the compensatory behaviors that characterize BN. In clinical samples, BED has generally been described among middle-aged men and women (the male to female ratio is approximately 2:3) who are overweight or obese. BED appears to affect a more an ethnically diverse subset of the population, unlike AN and BN, which occur among Caucasians much more frequently than among other ethnic groups.

Specific Features

The definition of binge-eating episodes associated with BED is identical in DSM-IV to the definition of such episodes in BN. However, the frequency criterion for BED is altered in two subtle ways. While the criteria for BN require a minimum average of two binge episodes per week for three 3 months, the criteria for BED require a minimum average of 2 days per week on which binge eating occurs over 6 months. Clinical experience and some objective data indicate that, during binges, individuals with BED consume a wider range of foods than do individuals with BN, whose binges are often confined to sweet, high-fat foods (Walsh &

Boudreau, 2003). Thus, the binge of a patient with BED more typically resembles a normal meal, except that it is much larger than normal in size. Another difference between individuals with BED and those with BN is that individuals with BED do not describe the extreme dietary restraint between binge eating episodes characteristic of BN. These differences in eating behavior highlight the importance of obtaining detailed information about eating habits during the evaluation.

Like individuals with AN and BN, individuals with BED express psychological concern regarding shape and weight, and the level of such concern is greater than that of similarly obese individuals without BED. Individuals with BED usually present for treatment not only because of a desire to stop binge eating, but also because they wish to lose a substantial amount of weight.

Medical Complications

BED is associated with significant medical morbidity, such as diabetes mellitus and hypertension, primarily related to the accompanying obesity (Bulik & Reichborn-Kjennerud, 2003).

Differential Diagnosis

Issues surrounding differential diagnosis are complicated by the uncertain status of BED in the psychiatric nomenclature. For example, the location of the boundary between BED and the nonpurging subtype of BN is unclear. Currently the distinction between nonpurging BN and BED hinges on an assessment of whether individuals' attempts to avoid weight gain are of sufficient frequency and inappropriateness to merit satisfying criteria for BN. Another disturbance characterized by binge eating and associated with obesity is night eating syndrome (NES), which is discussed later in this chapter. The characteristic difference between NES and BED is that, in NES, the overeating episodes occur primarily at night, including during awakenings from sleep (Birketvedt et al., 1999; Stunkard & Allison, 2003b). However, the literature comparing and contrasting the features of BED and NES is, as yet, modest.

As was noted regarding BN, major depression is sometimes associated with overeating, and a diagnosis of a mood disturbance should be considered when evaluating individuals with BED. In fact, a critical unresolved issue in the diagnostic nomenclature is whether BED would be better conceptualized as an indicator of mood disturbance among obese individuals (Stunkard & Allison, 2003a).

Eating Disorder Not Otherwise Specified

DSM-IV formally identifies only two eating disorders, AN and BN. All other clinically significant syndromes in which a disturbance of eating is the salient feature—including BED—are grouped in the broad and heterogeneous category of eating disorder not otherwise specified (EDNOS). In fact, a substantial fraction of individuals presenting for treatment of eating problems fall into this category.

Subthreshold Eating Disorders

Many individuals whose symptoms fall into EDNOS can reasonably be viewed as having subthreshold or atypical AN or BN. For example, this might include an individual who meets all the criteria for AN but who continues to menstruate, or an individual who meets all the criteria for BN but whose average frequency of binge eating and vomiting is only once per week over the last 3 months.

Night Eating Syndrome

A more distinct category within EDNOS is night eating syndrome (NES). NES is a disorder characterized by morning anorexia, evening hyperphagia, emotional distress, and insomnia, and may be viewed as a combination of an eating disorder, a sleep disorder, and a mood disorder. NES was originally described several decades ago, but has recently begun to receive increased attention (Stunkard & Allison, 2003b).

Childhood Eating Disorders

The description and study of eating disorders arising before puberty have received relatively little attention. However, there is no question about the potentially serious nature of behavioral abnormalities such as food refusal and idiosyncratic food selection, and investigators have recently begun to characterize such phenomena (Bryant-Waugh & Lask, 1995; Lask & Bryant-Waugh, 2000; Nicholls, Chater, & Lask, 2000).

SUMMARY

This chapter presented an overview of the essential components required in a thorough clinical assessment of individuals with eating disorders. To arrive at a valid diagnosis, the clinician should obtain a full description of the patient's eating behavior and the psychological and emotional concomitants of that behavior. The clinician should attempt to understand how these disturbances began and have evolved, and to estimate the patient's commitment to changing them. Other mental and general medical disorders that might account for some or all of the eating disturbances should be considered, and possible physical complications should be assessed. A thorough assessment should yield the likely diagnostic possibilities and provide a firm basis for treatment planning. Carrying out the assessment in a thorough but empathic fashion should also begin to build an alliance with the patient, which will increase the likelihood that treatment will be successful.

Finally, it should be noted that the assessment approach described in this chapter is a semistructured method that can be applied in most general clinical settings. A range of more structured assessment methods, both interview-based and self-report, are also available (Pike, Wolk, Gluck, & Walsh, 2000). These are routinely used in research settings, but may also be usefully employed in routine clinical practice to obtain more objective measures of the patient status.

REFERENCES

American Psychiatric Association. (1994). *Diagnostic and statistical manual of mental disorders* (4th ed.). Washington, DC: Author.

Beglin, S. J., & Fairburn, C. G. (1992). What is meant by the term "binge"? *American Journal of Psychiatry, 149*, 123–124.

Birketvedt, G. S., Florholmen, J., Sundsfjord, J., Osterud, B., Dinges, D., Bilker, W., & Stunkard, A. (1999). Behavioral and neuroendocrine characteristics of the night-eating syndrome. *Journal of the American Medical Association, 282*, 657–663.

Bryant-Waugh, R., & Lask, B. (1995). Eating disorders in children. *Journal of Child Psychology and Psychiatry and Allied Disciplines, 36*, 191–202.

Bulik, C. M., & Reichborn-Kjennerud, T. (2003). Medical morbidity in binge eating disorder. *International Journal of Eating Disorders, 34*(Suppl.), S39–S46.

Cachelin, F. M., & Maher, B. A. (1998). Is amenorrhea a critical criterion for anorexia nervosa? *Journal of Psychosomatic Research, 44*, 435–440.

Crow, S. J., Agras, W. S., Halmi, K., Mitchell, J. E., & Kraemer, H. C. (2002). Full syndromal versus subthreshold anorexia nervosa, bulimia nervosa, and binge eating disorder: A multicenter study. *International Journal of Eating Disorders, 32*, 209–318.

DaCosta, M., & Halmi, K. A. (1992). Classifications of anorexia nervosa: Question of subtypes. *International Journal of Eating Disorders, 11*, 305–313.

Garfinkel, P. E., Lin, E., Goering, P., Spegg, C., Goldbloom, D., Kennedy, S., Kaplan,

A. S., & Woodside, D. B. (1996a). Should amenorrhea be necessary for the diagnosis of anorexia nervosa? Evidence from a Canadian community sample. *British Journal of Psychiatry*, *168*, 500–506.

Garfinkel, P. E., Lin, E., Goering, P., Spegg, C., Goldbloom, D., Kennedy, S., Kaplan, A. S., & Woodside, D. B. (1996b). Purging and nonpurging forms of bulimia nervosa in a community sample. *International Journal of Eating Disorders*, *20*(3), 231–238.

Gleaves, D. H., Williamson, D. A., & Barker, S. E. (1993). Additive effects of mood and eating forbidden foods upon the perceptions of overeating and binging in bulimia nervosa. *Addictive Behaviors*, *18*, 299–309.

Halsted, C. H. (2001). Malnutrition and nutritional assessment. In E. Braunwald, A. S. Fauci, D. L. Kasper, S. L. Hauser, D. L. Longo, & J. L. Jameson (Eds.), *Harrison's principles of internal medicine* (15th ed., pp. 455–461). New York: McGraw-Hill.

Lask, B., & Bryant-Waugh, R. (Eds.). (2000). *Anorexia nervosa and related eating disorders in childhood and adolescence* (2nd ed.). Hove, UK: Psychology Press.

Metropolitan Life Insurance Company. (1983). 1983 height and weight tables for men and women. *Statistical Bulletin*, pp. 2–9.

Nicholls, D., Chater, R., & Lask, B. (2000). Children into DSM don't go: A comparison of classification systems for eating disorders in childhood and early adolescence. *International Journal of Eating Disorders*, *28*, 317–324.

Pike, K. M., Wolk, S. L., Gluck, M., & Walsh, B. T. (2000). Eating disorders measures. In American Psychiatric Association, *Handbook of psychiatric measures* (pp. 647–671). Washington, DC: American Psychiatric Association.

Stunkard, A. J., & Allison, K. C. (2003a). Binge eating disorder: Disorder or marker? *International Journal of Eating Disorders*, *34*(Suppl.), S107–S116.

Stunkard, A. J., & Allison, K. C. (2003b). Two forms of disordered eating in obesity: Binge eating and night eating. *International Journal of Obesity and Related Metabolic Disorders*, *27*, 1–12.

Walsh, B. T. (2001). Eating disorders. In E. Braunwald, A. S. Fauci, D. L. Kasper, S. L. Hauser, D. L. Longo, & J. L. Jameson (Eds.), *Harrison's principles of internal medicine* (15th ed., pp. 486–490). New York: McGraw-Hill.

Walsh, B. T., & Boudreau, G. (2003). Laboratory studies of binge eating disorder. *International Journal of Eating Disorders*, *34*(Suppl.), S30–S38.

Watson, T. L., & Andersen, A. E. (2003). A critical examination of the amenorrhea and weight criteria for diagnosing anorexia nervosa. *Acta Psychiatrica Scandinavica*, *108*, 175–182.

World Health Organization. (1992). *The ICD-10 classification of mental and behavioural disorders: Clinical descriptions and diagnostic guidelines*. Geneva, Switzerland: Author.

CHAPTER 2

The Classification of Eating Disorders

Kathryn H. Gordon
Jill M. Denoma
Thomas E. Joiner, Jr.

Human beings have a proclivity to classify everything that exists in the world around them. At a fundamental level, this propensity facilitates survival. At a more advanced level, it satisfies the need to recognize patterns, establish order, and enable communication. For scientists, classification is a crucial component in the pursuit of understanding and predicting events. To the degree that we are able to classify phenomena accurately, we will be able to gain a more precise understanding of the world around us, and an ability to predict future endeavors.

It is a challenging task to develop a classification scheme that accurately reflects the nature of psychopathology. Developing a classification system that represents the true nature of eating disorders begins with the accurate operationalization and description of these syndromes. Deeper understanding of the constructs that underlie eating disorders will help scientists create more precise theories about their nature. Accurate theories, in turn, will allow us to derive valid inferences that can be applied to populations of interest. Specifically, the value of creating an accurate classification system is that it will allow us to more successfully assess and recognize eating disorders, predict their onset and course, and understand what treatments work best for a given disorder.

DSM CLASSIFICATION OF EATING DISORDERS

Researchers and clinicians have perpetually struggled to develop a classification system that genuinely reflects the nature of psychopathology in general, and eating disorders in particular. As successive volumes of the *Diagnostic and Statistical Manual of Mental Disorders* (DSM) have been published, a variety of classification schemes have been employed. Currently, the DSM reflects a primarily descriptive system based upon clustering symptoms of psychopathological disorders. Of interest in this context is that the DSM has heavily influenced our conceptual models of and treatments for eating disorders. Presently, our classification system—based upon the DSM-IV-TR (the fourth edition, text revision, of the *Diagnostic and Statistical Manual of Mental Disorders*; American Psychiatric Association, 2000)—assumes qualitative distinctions between three main categories of eating disorders: anorexia nervosa (AN), bulimia nervosa (BN), and eating disorder not otherwise specified (EDNOS). Within the first two categories, DSM-IV-TR suggests that further subdivision is warranted, and it has consequently further divided the diagnostic categories into subtypes. In addition, DSM-IV-TR recognizes binge eating disorder (BED) in its appendix, although someone with its presentation would currently be given a diagnosis of EDNOS.

AN is characterized by a refusal to maintain a minimally normal body weight (defined as a weight less than 85% of that expected), an intense fear of gaining weight, and significant disturbance in body shape or size. In females, it is also accompanied by amenorrhea. When diagnosing someone with AN, a clinician is required to specify whether the client is a restricting subtype or binge–purge subtype. The restricting subtype is reserved for anorexics who lose weight primarily by dieting, fasting, or exercising. Furthermore, they do not regularly engage in binge eating or purging behaviors, while people classified in the binge–purge subtype do.

The second eating disorder presented in the DSM-IV-TR is BN. BN is diagnosed when someone engages in recurrent episodes of binge eating (characterized by consuming a very large amount of food in a discrete time period) and recurrent compensatory behaviors in order to prevent weight gain at an average frequency of twice per week for at least 3 months. Additionally, to be diagnosed with BN, a person's body shape and weight must unduly influence self-evaluations. The DSM-IV-TR specifies that this disorder cannot be diagnosed if it occurs exclusively during episodes of AN. Once a diagnosis of BN is given, a clinician must specify whether the person meets criteria for the purging or nonpurging subtype.

People who are diagnosed with the purging subtype are those that regularly engage in self-induced vomiting or the misuse of laxatives, diuretics, or enemas. People who meet criteria for the nonpurging type are those that regularly use inappropriate compensatory behaviors such as fasting or excessive exercise, but not vomiting or laxatives, to control their weight.

Finally, the EDNOS category is reserved for people who exhibit many of the characteristics common in other eating disorders and have a clinically significant eating disorder syndrome, but whose symptoms deviate from those specified in the AN and BN diagnostic criteria. One reason for such a diagnosis is a subclinical level of symptomatology for AN or BN. Examples of people who may qualify for this diagnosis are females who meet all qualifications for AN except the loss of menses, or people who meet all qualifications for BN except that the frequency of their bingeing and purging is slightly less than twice a week or has been occurring for less than 3 months.

It is important to note that BED is currently classified as an example of EDNOS, although it is more explicitly described in the DSM-IV-TR appendix. Because the DSM-IV eating disorders task force (the task force was for DSM-IV, not DSM-IV-TR) recommended that the possibility of BED existing as a separate diagnostic entity be researched, they have set forth potential diagnostic criteria to be examined. People who experience recurrent episodes of binge eating in the absence of regular use of inappropriate compensatory behaviors are given a diagnosis of EDNOS, and typically referred to as having BED. Symptomatically, people with BED may experience a sense of loss of control when consuming large amounts of food, feel distress when bingeing, eat more rapidly than usual, eat when they are not hungry, eat until uncomfortably full, eat alone due to embarrassment about overeating, and/or feel disgusted with themselves for overeating.

Research has demonstrated some reliable differences in symptom presentations between people diagnosed with AN, BN, and BED. One clear example is the fact that people diagnosed with AN are severely underweight, while those diagnosed with BN are often of an average weight (Johnson, Stuckey, Lewis, & Schwartz, 1982) and those with BED are typically overweight (Spitzer et al., 1992). There is also evidence of demographic differences among people diagnosed with the different eating disorders. While women are more likely to be diagnosed with eating disorders than men, the proportion of females to males varies between diagnostic entities. Both AN and BN occur at approximately a 9:1 or 10:1 ratio of females to males, whereas BED occurs at approximately a 3:2 ratio (Spitzer et al., 1992). Additionally, it seems that people with BED are older, on average, than those with BN. For example, in one study by Masheb and Grilo (2000), people with BED were 43.6 (*SD* = 9) years old, while those with BN were 31.8 (*SD* = 10) years old. Finally, it is apparent that people diagnosed with AN are at the greatest risk for mortality. It is estimated that more than 10% of anorexics will die from this disorder, while mortality rates for other eating disorders are significantly lower (Quadflieg & Fichter, 2003).

Despite the existence of three unique categories of eating disorders, previous researchers have identified psychological, physiological, and personality characteristics that transcend diagnostic boundaries. By definition, there are cognitive and behavioral components common to some of the eating disorders. For instance, individuals diagnosed with AN, BN, and BED all put an undue amount of influence on their body shape or size when engaging in self-evaluative processes (Fairburn, 1995). Furthermore, they feel compelled to go to extreme, inappropriate lengths in an effort to prevent weight gain. People diagnosed with both BED and BN engage in periods of binge eating, during which they feel a lack of control over eating behaviors. Additionally, people diagnosed with the binge–purge subtype of AN engage in periods of binge eating that are similar to those experienced by people with BN or BED.

Certain psychological variables also frequently exist across eating disorder diagnoses. For example, it has been reported that people diagnosed with AN and BN both experience high rates of comorbidity with mood, anxiety, substance use, and personality disorders (Wonderlich & Mitchell, 1997). Recently, it has been demonstrated that people diagnosed with BED also experience high rates of mood disorders, anxiety disorders, and suicidal symptoms (Johnson, Spitzer, & Williams, 2001). Additionally, there appears to be an increased rate of eating, mood, and anxiety disorders in the families of patients with BED (Fairburn, Doll, Welch, Hay, Davies, & O'Connor, 1998), BN (Garfinkel et al., 1996), and AN (Rivinus et al., 1984; Bulik, 1995), which may suggest that these disorders may share a common genetic diathesis. Also of interest is the frequent crossover between the diagnostic categories of eating disorders, which raises questions about their independence. Specifically, many people of normal weight diagnosed with BN have a history of AN, and most people diagnosed with AN will ultimately develop symptoms associated with BN (Keel, Mitchell, Davis, Fieselman, & Crow, 2000; Herzog et al., 1999). Thus, there seems to be considerable diagnostic heterogeneity within the categories of AN, BN, and BED, which is highlighted by the high degree of psychological comorbidity and diagnostic crossover often observed in patients with eating disorders.

A variety of intrapersonal and interpersonal characteristics appear frequently in people suffering from eating disorders. For instance, it is very common for people with eating disorders to suffer from low self-esteem. This finding has been consistently reported in literature examining people with BN, AN (Gonzales, 2001), and BED (Fairburn, 1995). In addition, similarities appear in the psychosocial patterns of people with various eating disorders. Hsu et al. (2002) reported that individuals with BED experience a high degree of impairment in social functioning, while Gonzales (2001) reported a similar finding for people with AN. Likewise, social skills problems are reported both by women suffering from BN and by outside observers (Grisset & Norvell, 1992). Finally, self-perceived social skills deficits have been shown to predict the onset of future BN symptoms (Gordon, Otamendi, Joiner, Lewinsohn, & Keel, 2005). In sum, patients with eating disorders clearly present with significantly more negative interpersonal profiles compared to controls (Bjorck, Clinton, Sohlberg, Hallstrom, & Norring, 2003).

Neurotransmitter research suggests that serotonergic dysregulation (specifically, hyposerotonergic status) is associated with each of the eating disorders, as well. In individuals with AN, results have demonstrated decreased platelet binding of serotonin (5-hydroxytryptophan [5-HT]) uptake inhibitors (Weizman, Carmi, Tyano, Apter, & Rehavi, 1986), blunted prolactin and cortisol responses to 5-HT agonists and partial agonists (Monteleone, Brambrilla, Bortolototti, LaRocca, & Maj, 1998), and reduced cerebrospinal fluid levels of 5-HT metabolite (Kaye, Ebert, Raleight, & Lake, 1984). Similarly, individuals with BN tend to have decreased cerebrospinal fluid levels of 5-hydroxyindoleacetic acid (Jimerson, Lesem, Kaye, & Brewerton, 1992), reduced platelet binding of 5-HT uptake inhibitors (Marazitti, Macchi, Rotondo, Placidi, & Cassano, 1988), reduced central transport availability (Tauscher et al., 2001), and blunted neuroendocrine responses to 5-HT precursors and 5-HT agonists or partial agonists (Jimerson et al., 1992). Finally, women diagnosed with BED have been reported to have reduced 5-HT transporter binding (Kuikka et al., 2001). Thus current research demonstrates that women with each of the eating disorders experiences serotonergic dysregulation.

CLASSIFICATION OF EATING DISORDERS USING PERSONALITY TYPES

We have presented some research that supports the current DSM-IV-TR classification system of eating disorders, such as evidence that the average body weight, medical complications, and demographic characteristics differ between eating disorder diagnostic groups. However, we have also presented research that suggests substantial overlap and crossover of comorbid symptoms, psychological variables (e.g., low self-esteem), and serotonergic dysregulation across diagnostic categories. In addition, some research suggests substantial heterogeneity within eating disorder diagnostic categories that may not be captured by DSM-IV-TR subtypes. For example, the AN binge–purge type may be more accurately considered as a variation of BN. Similarly, there has been some debate over the validity of purging and nonpurging subtype distinction for BN (Gleaves, Lowe, Green, Cororve, & Williams, 2000; Williamson et al., 2002).

It has also been suggested that subtypes of eating disorder categories may be best classified according to personality characteristics (Wonderlich & Mitchell, 2001). Certain personality variables have been shown to cut across eating disorder diagnoses. Researchers have shown that impulsivity is common among individuals diagnosed with BN (Diaz-Marsa, Carrasco, & Saiz, 2000; Casper, Hedeker, & McClough, 1992; Williamson, Kelley, Davis, Ruggeiro & Blouin, 1985), AN (Fahy & Eisler, 1993), and BED (de Zwaan, et al., 1994; Hsu et al., 2002). Although restricting subtype anorexics are believed to be less impulsive than binge–purge subtype anorexics (Nagata, Kawarada, Kiriike, & Iketani, 2000), there is controversy regarding the existence of impulsivity in people with AN binge–purge subtype. Whereas Nagata et al. found evidence that individuals with AN purge subtype had many more multi-impulsive features than controls, Casper, Hedeker, and McClough (1992) reported that these types of patients tended to be in the low normal range of impulsivity. These contrasting findings may speak to the large within-subjects variability observed in patients with eating disorders. Narcissism has been identified as another personality variable that exists in individuals with either BN or AN (Steiger, Jabalpurwala, Champagne, & Stotland, 1997).

A series of cluster analytic studies have been conducted to evaluate the possibility that individuals with eating disorders can be grouped by personality characteristics. Three personality types have consistently emerged in these studies. First, Strober (1983) cluster analyzed Minnesota Multiphasic Personality Inventory (MMPI; Hathaway & McKinley, 1943) profiles of women diagnosed with AN and discerned three personality types: a high-functioning group with high levels of conformity and need for control; a socially avoidant and anxious, self-doubting group; and an impulsive group with poor coping strategies and a poor prognosis. In a similar study, Goldner, Srikameswaran, Schroeder, Livesley, and Birmingham (1999) cluster analyzed responses to the Dimensional Assessment of Personality Pathology

(DAPP; Livesley, Jackson, & Schroeder, 1991) and identified three groups: one that was similar to controls and exhibited minimal personality pathology; another with high levels of compulsivity and interpersonal difficulties; and a third who seemed psychopathic, neurotic, and impulsive. Interestingly, in the Goldner study, particular eating disorder diagnoses were not linked to specific personality-based clusters. Finally, Westen and Harnden-Fischer (2001) cluster analyzed the clinician Q-sorts of personality traits in patients with eating disorders and again found three categories of patients: a high-functioning, perfectionist group; a rigid and overcontrolled group; and an emotionally dysregulated and undercontrolled group. Important in the context of classification, these personality clusters have been associated with different patterns of etiological variables, symptomatic presentation, and level of adaptive functioning. Furthermore, several studies suggest that particular personality variables cut across eating disorder diagnoses and that variability within eating disorder categories is greater than between categories (Abbot, Wonderlich & Mitchell, 2001; Grilo et al., 2003; Westen & Harnden-Fischer, 2001; Wonderlich & Mitchell, 2001).

One personality-based organizational scheme that has been used in the area of eating disorders distinguishes multi-impulsive bulimics from uni-impulsive bulimics (Fichter, Quadflieg, & Rief, 1994; Lacey, 1993). As the name suggests, multi-impulsive bulimia is characterized by multiple forms of behavioral impulsivity beyond binge–purge behavior. For example, Fichter et al. (1994) found that bulimic women who reported at least three impulsive behaviors (i.e., suicide attempts, self-harm, stealing, severe alcohol abuse, sexual promiscuity, drug abuse) exhibited more general psychopathology symptoms, and tended to have a worse course of illness than bulimic women without multiple impulsive behaviors (Fichter et al., 1994; Wiederman & Pryor, 1996). Research regarding the base rates of multi-impulsive bulimia has yielded mixed results. Welch and Fairburn (1996) found that multi-impulsive bulimia occurred at a low rate among bulimic women. However, Crosby et al. (2001) found that approximately 40% of bulimic individuals display at least three forms of destructive impulsive behaviors. Research examining the severity of eating disorder symptoms in the multi-impulsive groups has similarly yielded unclear results, where multi-impulsive bulimics appear to have more severe symptoms than their uni-impulsive counterparts on some measures, and equivalent severity on other measures (Fahy & Eisler, 1993; Wiederman & Pryor, 1996). Less research has been conducted regarding the prevalence of multiple forms of impulsivity in AN, but rates of multi-impulsivity appear higher in the binge–purge type than in the restricting type (Nagata et al., 2000).

Important with regards to classification system utility, the personality type of individuals with eating disorders appears to be related to treatment outcome (Mitchell, Crosby, Wonderlich, Myers, & Swan-Kremeier, 2003). Borderline personality disorder, DSM-IV-TR Cluster B personality disorders, and impulsivity are linked with poorer outcomes in individual and group therapy (Herzog, Keller, Lavori, & Sacks, 1991), cognitive-behavioral therapy (Rossiter, Agras, Telch, & Schneider, 1993), and pharmacotherapy (Rossiter et al., 1993). Also, individuals with comorbid eating disorders and Cluster B or borderline personality disorders show more general psychopathology, substance use, self-destructive behavior, suicide attempts, histories of sexual or physical abuse, and negative appraisals of family functioning, greater hospitalization rates, and higher utilization of psychotropic medication than other individuals with eating disorders (Johnson, Tobin, & Dennis, 1990; Steiger & Stotland, 1996; Wonderlich & Swift, 1990).

CLASSIFICATION OF EATING DISORDERS USING TAXOMETRICS

Schmidt, Kotov, and Joiner (2004) stated that classification systems serve two important functions. First, they should be useful organizational systems by which we meaningfully group information. The DSM has advanced the field of psychopathology by allowing a system for which clinicians and researchers can communicate through standard definitions of disorders. This service, alone, makes the DSM classification system worthwhile. However, another important factor is desirable in a classification system—that it accurately represent nature rather than be an arbitrary grouping system. The DSM assumes a categorical nature of psychiatric disorders (that is, a person either has a disorder or does not, rather than falling somewhere on a continuum). However, the DSM acknowledges that this approach has limitations, and that certain disorders may be more accurately conceived of as occurring dimensionally. Thus, it is possible that the DSM may not accurately represent nature in its current form. An accurate classification system is essential to the advance of science, because it serves as a springboard for valid research. Properly identifying and conceptualizing psychiatric disorders is the most efficient and precise way to design studies that further our understanding of such phenomena and enable us to confidently interpret findings as meaningful (Schmidt et al., 2004).

Taxometric methodologies are data-analytic tools designed specifically to address questions about the latent structure of phenomena in nature (i.e. taxon or continuum; Waller & Meehl, 1998). Taxometrics, therefore, can be very useful in assessing the accuracy of classification system conceptualizations of psychiatric disorders. For example, regarding eating disorders, taxometric analyses could directly speak to the debate over whether AN and BN are actually qualitatively separate classes (which would imply a taxon) or different manifestations of the same disorder (which would imply a continuum). Furthermore, taxometrics could be used to determine the existence of subtypes within taxon membership. For example, are individuals with the nonpurging vs. the purging subtype of bulimia qualitatively different?

A small group of taxometric studies have addressed the latent nature of eating disorders. More research has been conducted on BN, likely due to higher base rates of BN than AN (Schmidt et al., 2004). Gleaves, Lowe, Snow, Green, and Murphy-Eberenz (2000) conducted the first taxometric study of eating disorders. They examined the latent structure of BN in a mixed sample of undergraduates and participants recruited from an eating disorder clinic, and found evidence of a latent taxon for BN. It is worth noting that some have criticized this study, saying that the latent taxon may have emerged as an artifact of using a mixed population (Tylka & Subich, 2003).

Williamson et al. (2002) conducted a taxometric analysis examining all the DSM-IV-TR eating disorder diagnoses. The sample included a clinical group diagnosed with eating disorders (BN, AN, BED, and EDNOS), nonclinical undergraduates, and obese participants. Their results provided support that eating disorders are best conceptualized as a latent taxon. Furthermore, they provided evidence that BN and BED are best represented as discrete entities, while AN may occur on a continuum. Finally, they proposed that AN binge–purge subtype, BED, and BN (eating disorders that involve bingeing) are a distinct class, qualitatively different from AN. Here again, the results should be interpreted with caution because the study included methodological problems such as incomplete reporting of the analyses and the base rates, as well as small sample sizes for the diagnostic groups (Schmidt et al., 2004).

Tylka and Subich (2003) conducted a study that challenged the discontinuity findings for eating disorders. Using a large sample of college-aged women, they found results suggesting that the latent structure of eating disorders is dimensional rather than taxonic. Limitations to their study include sole use of self-report measures and the exclusion of any behavioral indicators (such as bingeing or purging). In sum, two of the three taxometric studies (Gleaves, Lowe, Snow, et al., 2000; Williamson et al., 2002) suggest that BN is taxonic in nature, which suggests that it is qualitatively different from milder forms of eating disturbances. So far, the AN restricting type does not appear to be taxonic in nature when compared to less extreme forms of eating disturbances (e.g., chronic dieting; Williamson et al., 2002). Finally, BED appears to be a discrete entity, separate from both normal weight and obese nonbinge eating participants (Williamson et al., 2002).

Taxometric studies have also examined the DSM subtypes of eating disorders. Gleaves, Lowe, Green, et al. (2000) and Williamson et al. (2002) found support that AN-restricting subtype is qualitatively distinct from the AN binge–purge subtype, and that AN binge–purge subtype is not qualitatively distinct from BN. These findings suggest that AN binge–purge subtype might be more appropriately grouped with BN rather than AN-restricting type in future editions of the DSM.

SUMMARY

In conclusion, the current DSM-IV-TR classification system has been useful in the assessment, treatment, and scientific study of eating disorders. It has provided an organizational structure and facilitated communication between clinicians and researchers. However, an ideal classification system accurately reflects nature as well. The DSM-IV-TR may not completely satisfy this criterion. The extant literature base indicates heterogeneity within DSM diagnostic categories and subtypes, as well as similarities across DSM diagnostic categories (beyond the mere presence of disturbed eating).

Cluster analytic studies suggest that individuals with eating disorders might be better classified into subtypes that reflect personality traits rather than differentiating through eating symptoms. Taxometrics is an ideal way to test whether or not personality characteristic types among the eating disorders represent truly distinct classes. To date, no studies have been conducted that test the idea that highly impulsive forms of eating disorders (e.g., multi-impulsive bulimia, comorbid borderline personality disorder) represent a true taxon or a class of individuals with eating disorders that is qualitatively different from uni-impulsive or compulsive forms of eating disorders. This may be of particular importance considering findings that patients with eating disorders and comorbid Cluster B personality disorders tend to have poor prognoses (Johnson et al., 1990; Steiger & Stotland, 1996; Wonderlich & Swift, 1990). Future studies in this area may reveal alternative conceptualizations to the current DSM classification system.

Taxometric analyses have revealed that eating disorders might be more accurately classified as those involving bingeing (e.g., BED, BN, and AN binge–purge subtype, subclinical BN) versus restricting types (AN restricting type, subclinical AN). Additional taxometric analyses that address methodological concerns in existing research are needed to test the validity of earlier findings and current DSM categories. Furthermore, taxometric studies examining the diagnostic category of EDNOS would clarify if there is a qualitative difference between subclinical eating disorders and full syndrome eating disorders. Considering the fact that no significant clinical or demographic differences emerge between clinical and subclinical BN (Kendler, Maclean, & Neale, 1991), this study could be of particular import to future versions of the DSM. Finally, at least one taxometric study (Williamson et al., 2002) supports BED as a discrete diagnostic category, which suggests that it may be appropriate to move it from the appendix into the eating disorders section of the DSM.

Finally, future taxometric studies including genetic, biological, and family characteristics as indicators may shed light on diagnostic grouping issues, as they have the potential to reveal which disorders might share genetic diatheses. This kind of work has the potential to inform etiological models of eating disorders, and may eventually give rise to effective prevention strategies. Ultimately, longitudinal studies are needed to determine the predictive validity and utility of diagnostic categories. Longitudinal studies may serve to inform the course, treatment choice, and theory underlying eating disorders. Future refinement of the DSM classification system through the use of tools such as taxometrics may serve as a springboard for more precise identification, assessment, understanding, and treatment of eating disorders.

REFERENCES

Abbott, D. W., Wonderlich, S. A., & Mitchell, J. E. (2001). Treatment implications of comorbid personality disorders. In J. E. Mitchell (Ed.), *The outpatient treatment of eating disorders: A guide for therapists, dietitians, and physicians*. Minneapolis: University of Minnesota Press.

American Psychiatric Association. (2000). *Diagnostic and statistical manual of mental disorders* (4th ed., text rev.). Washington, DC: Author.

Bjorck, C., Clinton, D., Sohlberg, S., Hallstrom, T., & Norring, C. (2003). Interpersonal profiles in eating disorders: Ratings of SASB self-image. *Psychology & Psychotherapy: Theory, Research & Practice, 76*(4), 337–349.

Bulik, C. M. (1995). Anxiety disorders and eating disorders: A review of their relationship. *New Zealand Journal of Psychology, 24*(2), 51–62.

Casper, R. C., Hedeker, D., & McClough, J. F. (1992). Personality dimensions in eating disorders and their relevance for subtyping. *Journal of the American Academy of Child and Adolescent Psychiatry, 31*(5), 830–840.

Crosby, R. D., Wonderlich, S. A., Redlin, J., Engel, S. G., Simonich, H., Jones-Paxton, M., et al. (2001, November). *Impulsive behavior patterns in a sample of females with bulimia nervosa.* Poster presented at the annual meeting of the Eating Disorders Research Society, Bernalillo, NM.

de Zwaan, M., Mitchell, J. E., Seim, H. C., Specker, S. M., Pyle R. L., Raymond, M., & Crosby, R. B. (1994). Eating related and general psychopathology in obese females with binge eating disorder. *International Journal of Eating Disorders, 15*(1), 43–52.

Diaz-Marsa, M., Carrasco, J. L., & Saiz, J. (2000). A study of temperament and personality in anorexia and bulimia nervosa. *Journal of Personality Disorders, 14*(4), 352–359.

Fahy, T. A., & Eisler, I. (1993). Impulsivity and eating disorders. *British Journal of Psychiatry, 162*, 193–197.

Fairburn, C. G. (1995). *Overcoming binge eating.* New York: Guilford Press.

Fairburn, C. G., Doll, H. A., Welch, S. L., Hay, P. J., Davies, B. A., & O'Connor, M. E. (1998). Risk factors for binge eating disorder: A community-based, case-control study. *Archives of General Psychiatry, 55*, 425–432.

Fichter, M. M., Quadflieg, N., & Rief, W. (1994). Course of multi-impulsive bulimia. *Psychological Medicine, 24*, 591–604.

Garfinkel, P. E., Lin, E., Goering, P., Spegg, C., Goldbloom, D. S., Kennedy, S., Kaplan, A. S., & Woodside, D. B. (1996). Purging and nonpurging forms of bulimia nervosa in a community sample. *International Journal of Eating Disorders, 20*(3), 231–238.

Gleaves, D. H., Lowe, M. R., Green, B. A., Cororve, M. B., & Williams, T. L. (2000). Do anorexia and bulimia nervosa occur on a continuum? A taxometric analysis. *Behavior Therapy, 31*, 195–219.

Gleaves, D. H., Lowe, M. R., Snow, A. C., Green, B. A., & Murphy-Eberenz, K. P. (2000). Continuity and discontinuity models of bulimia nervosa: A taxometric investigation. *Journal of Abnormal Psychology, 109*(1), 56–68.

Goldner, E. M., Srikameswaran, S., Schroeder, M. L., Livesley, W. J., & Birmingham, C. L. (1999). Dimensional assessment of personality pathology in patients with eating disorders. *Psychiatry Research, 85*, 151–159.

Gonzales, E. G. (2001). Evaluation of self-concept, body satisfaction and social skills in anorexia and bulimia nervosa. *Clínica y Salud, 12*(3), 289–304.

Gordon, K. H., Otamendi, A., Joiner, T. E., Jr., Lewinsohn, P. M., & Keel, P. K. (2005). *Self-perceived social skills deficits and negative life events interact to predict the onset of bulimia nervosa symptoms.* Manuscript submitted for publication.

Grilo, C. M., Sanislow, C. A., Skodol, A. E., Gunderson, J. G., Sout, R. L., Shea, M. T., et al. (2003). Do eating disorders co-occur with personality disorders? Comparison groups matter. *International Journal of Eating Disorders, 33*, 155–164.

Grisset, N. I., & Norvell, N. K. (1992). Perceived social support, social skills, and quality of relationships in bulimic women. *Journal of Consulting and Clinical Psychology*, 60, 293–299.

Hathaway, S. R., & McKinley, J. C. (1943). *The Minnesota Multiphasic Personality Inventory*. Minneapolis: University of Minnesota Press.

Herzog, D. B., Dorer, D. J., Keel, P. K., Swleyn, S. E., Ekeblad, E. R., Flores, A. T., et al. (1999). Recovery and relapse in anorexia and bulimia: A 7.5-year follow-up study. *Journal of the American Academy of Child and Adolescent Psychiatry, 38*(7), 829–837.

Herzog, D. B., Keller, M. B., Lavori, P. W., & Sacks, N. R. (1991). The course and outcome of bulimia nervosa. *Journal of Clinical Psychiatry, 52*(Suppl.), 4–8.

Hsu, L. K. G., Mulliken, B., McDonagh, B., Das, S. K., Rand, W., Fairburn, C. G., et al. (2002). Binge eating disorder in extreme obesity. *International Journal of Obesity and Related Metabolic Disorders, 26*(10), 1398–1403.

Jimerson, D. C., Lesem, M. D., Kaye, W. H., & Brewerton, T. D. (1992). Low serotonin and dopamine metabolite concentration in cerebrospinal fluid from bulimic patients with frequent binge episodes. *Archives of General Psychiatry, 49*, 132–138.

Johnson, C. L., Stuckey, M. K., Lewis, L. D., & Schwartz, D. M. (1982). Bulimia: A descriptive study of 316 cases. *International Journal of Eating Disorders, 2*(1), 3–16.

Johnson, C. L., Tobin, D. L., & Dennis, A. (1990). Differences in treatment outcome between borderline and non-borderline bulimics at one year follow-up. *International Journal of Eating Disorders*, 9, 617–627.

Johnson, J. G., Spitzer, R. L., & Williams, B. W. (2001). Health problems, impairment, and illnesses associated with bulimia nervosa and binge eating disorder among primary care and obstetric gynaecology patients. *Psychological Medicine, 31*, 1455–1466.

Kaye, W. H., Ebert, M. H., Raleigh, M., & Lake, R. (1984). Abnormalities in CNS monoamine metabolism in anorexia nervosa. *Archives of General Psychiatry, 41*, 350–355.

Keel, P. K., Mitchell, J. E., Davis, T. L., Fieselman, S., & Crow, S. J. (2000). Impact of definitions on the description and prediction of bulimia nervosa outcome. *International Journal of Eating Disorders, 28*, 377–386.

Kendler, K. S., Maclean, C., & Neale, M. (1991). The genetic epidemiology of bulimia nervosa. American Journal of Psychiatry, 148, 1627–1637.

Kuikka, J. T., Tammela, L., Karhunen, L., Rissanen, A., Bergstrom, K. A., Naukkarinen, H., et al. (2001). Reduced serotonin transporter binding in binge eating women. *Psychopharmacology, 155*, 310–314.

Lacey, J. H. (1993). Self-damaging and addictive behaviour in bulimia nervosa: A catchment area study. *British Journal of Psychiatry, 163*, 190–194.

Livesley, W. J., Jackson, D. N., & Schroeder, M. L. (1991). Dimensions of personality pathology. *Canadian Journal of Psychiatry, 36*, 557–562.

Marazitti, D., Macchi, E., Rotondo, A., Placidi, G. F., & Cassano, G. B. (1988). Involvement of the serotonin system in bulimia. *Life Sciences, 43*, 2123–2126.

Masheb, R. M., & Grilo, C. M. (2000). Binge eating disorder: A need for additional diagnostic criteria. *Comprehensive Psychiatry, 41*(3), 159–162.

Mitchell, J. E., Crosby, R. D., Wonderlich, S. A., Myers, T., & Swan-Kremeier, L. (2003, September). *The influence of comorbidity on treatment response and prognosis in patients with bulimia nervosa.* Paper presented at the 9th Annual Meeting of the Eating Disorder Research Society, Ravello, Italy.

Monteleone, P., Brambrilla, F., Bortolototti, F., LaRocca, A., & Maj, M. (1998). Prolactin response to d-fenfluramine is blunted in people with anorexia nervosa. *British Journal of Psychiatry, 172*, 438–442.

Nagata, T., Kawarada, Y., Kiriike, N., & Iketani, T. (2000). Multi-impulsivity of Japanese patients with eating disorders: Primary and secondary impulsivity. *Psychiatry Research, 94*(3), 239–250.

Quadflieg, N., & Fichter, M. M. (2003). The course and outcome of bulimia nervosa. *European Child and Adolescent Psychiatry, 12*(Suppl. 1), i99-i109.

Rivinus, T. M., Biederman, J., Herzog, D. B., Kemper, K., Harper, G. P., Harmatz, J. S., & Houseworth, S. (1984). Anorexia nervosa and affective disorders: A controlled family history study. *American Journal of Psychiatry, 141*(11), 1414–1418.

Rossiter, E. M., Agras, W. S., Telch, C. F., & Schneider, J. A. (1993). Cluster B personality disorder characteristics predict outcome in treatment of bulimia nervosa. *International Journal of Eating Disorders, 13*, 349–357.

Schmidt, N. B., Kotov, R., & Joiner, T. E., Jr. (2004). Taxometrics: Toward a new diagnostic scheme for psychopathology. Washington, DC: American Psychological Association.

Spitzer, R. L, Devlin, M. J., Walsh, T. B., Hasin, D., Wing, R., Marcus, M., et al. (1992). Binge eating disorder: A multisite field trial of the diagnostic criteria. *International Journal of Eating Disorders, 11*(3), 191–203.

Steiger, H., & Stotland, S. (1996). Prospective study of outcome in bulimics as a function of Axis-II comorbidity: Long-term responses on eating and psychiatric symptoms. *International Journal of Eating Disorders, 20*, 149–162.

Steiger, H., Jabalpurwala, S., Champagne, J., & Stotland, S. (1997). A controlled study of trait narcissism in anorexia and bulimia nervosa. *International Journal of Eating Disorders, 22*(2), 173–178.

Strober, M. (1983). An empirically derived typology of anorexia nervosa. In P. L. Darby, P. E. Garfinkel, D. M. Garner, & D. V. Coscina (Eds.), *Anorexia nervosa: Recent developments in research.* New York: Liss.

Tauscher, J., Pirker, W., Willeit, M., de Zwaan, M., Bailer, U., Neumeister, A., et al. (2001). Beta-CIT and single photon emission computer tomography reveal reduced brain serotonin transporter availability in bulimia nervosa. *Biological Psychiatry, 49*, 326–332.

Tylka, T. L., & Subich, L. M. (2003). Revisiting the latent structure of eating disorders: Taxometric analyses with nonbehavioral indicators. *Journal of Counseling Psychology, 50*(3), 276–286.

Waller, N. G., & Meehl, P. E. (1998). *Multivariate taxometric procedures: Distinguishing types from continua.* Newbury Park, CA: Sage.

Weizman, R., Carmi, M., Tyano, S., Apter, A., & Rehavi, M. (1986). High affinity [–3H]imipramine binding and serotonin uptake to platelets of adolescent females suffering from anorexia nervosa. Life Sciences, 38, 1235–1242.

Welch, S. L., & Fairburn, C. G. (1996). Impulsivity or comorbidity in bulimia nervosa: A controlled study of deliberate self-harm and alcohol and drug misuse in a community sample. *British Journal of Psychiatry, 169*, 451–458.

Westen, D., & Harnden-Fischer, J. (2001). Personality profiles in eating disorders: Rethinking the distinction between Axis I and Axis II. *American Journal of Psychiatry, 158*, 547–562.

Wiederman, M. W., & Pryor, T. (1996). Multi-impulsivity among women with BN. *International Journal of Eating Disorders, 20*, 359–365.

Williamson, D. A., Womble, L. G., Smeets, M. A. M., Netemeyer, R. G., Thaw, J. M., Kutlesic, V., et al. (2002). Latent structure of eating disorder symptoms: A factor analytic and taxometric investigation. *American Journal of Psychiatry, 159*, 412–418.

Williamson, D. A., Kelley, M. L., Davis, C. J., Ruggeiro, L., & Blouin, D. (1985). Psychopathology of eating: A controlled comparison of bulimic, obese, and normal subjects. *Journal of Consulting and Clinical Psychology, 53*, 161–166.

Wonderlich, S. A., & Mitchell, J. E. (1997). Eating disorders and comorbidity: Empirical, conceptual, and clinical implications. *Psychopharmacology Bulletin, 33*, 381–390.

Wonderlich, S. A., & Mitchell, J. E. (2001). The role of personality in the onset of eating disorders and treatment implications. *Psychiatric Clinics of North America: Eating Disorders, 24*, 249–258.

Wonderlich, S. A., & Swift, W. J. (1990). Borderline versus other personality disorders in the eating disorders: Clinical description. *International Journal of Eating Disorders*, 9(6), 629–638.

CHAPTER 3

Conducting the Diagnostic Interview

Carol B. Peterson

Diagnostic interviewing is crucial to both clinical work and research with patients with eating disorders. Clinically, diagnostic interviewing facilitates treatment planning and provides information about the likelihood of course and outcome. In addition, the interview process can build rapport and provide a foundation for the therapeutic relationship. In research, diagnostic accuracy is essential to the quality of the data and the interpretation of results. Clinicians and researchers both benefit from accurate diagnoses by identifying the symptoms, medical risks, and comorbidity associated with each type of eating disorder as well as specific subtypes. For example, understanding whether a patient meets criteria for the restricting or the binge–purge type of anorexia nervosa (AN) provides the clinician with valuable information about potential psychiatric and medical comorbidity.

Although diagnostic interviewing is critically important, it is also challenging for a number of reasons. Patients often report difficulty remembering their symptoms accurately. Cognitive biases can result in erroneous recall of thoughts, feelings, and behaviors (Schacter, 1999). Patients with eating disorders can be particularly difficult to diagnose because some may minimize their symptoms in an effort to avoid treatment, or they may lack the self-awareness to be able to answer certain questions (Anderson & Paulosky, 2004; Vitousek, Daly, & Heiser, 1991). A number of eating disorder symptoms are also difficult to assess because of the complexity of the phenomena. For example, the undue influence of shape and weight on self-evaluation, included in the DSM-IV-TR criteria (American Psychiatric Association, 2000) for both AN and bulimia nervosa (BN), is a complicated concept that requires patients to have both the self-awareness and the abstract reasoning ability to identify how they determine their self-evaluation.

This chapter discusses specific strategies for conducting diagnostic interviewing with patients with eating disorders. The introductory section focuses on rapport and provides a brief review of standard interviews that can be used to diagnose eating disorder symptoms. The second section describes specific strategies to evaluate various diagnostic features of eating disorders. The third section provides information about other aspects of diagnostic interviewing with eating disorder patients, including comorbid psychopathology. Specific diagnostic issues related to the criteria for eating disorders, as well as strategies for making differential diagnoses, are described in detail in Chapter 1.

ESTABLISHING RAPPORT

The importance of rapport in diagnostic interviewing cannot be overemphasized. Whether the interview is conducted in a clinical or research setting, good rapport between the patient and interviewer is absolutely essential for several reasons. First, the establishment of rapport helps ensure that interactions between the interviewer and the patient are respectful. Second, the early development of rapport can establish the foundation for an ongoing relationship, which is especially important in treatment settings but can also be a consideration in research settings. Third, good rapport will improve the quality of information or data provided by the patient. If the interviewer does not work to establish a respectful and collaborative working relationship, the patient will be more hesitant to reveal personal information.

Establishing rapport can be particularly difficult with patients with eating disorders, especially with those who are ambivalent or even hostile about being interviewed. One of the most challenging tasks for the clinician is to remain patient even when the person being interviewed is withdrawn or angry. When conducted skillfully, a diagnostic interviewing can actually increase the patient's willingness to engage in the discussion because it enables the interviewer to demonstrate through questioning a clear grasp of the patient's subjective experience. Because patients with eating disorders often feel isolated, ashamed, and confused about their symptoms, empathetic questioning that reveals a thorough understanding about thoughts, feelings, and behaviors can facilitate an alliance between the patient and the interviewer. For example:

INTERVIEWER: Can you tell me some more about your eating patterns?

PATIENT: Like what?

INTERVIEWER: Perhaps you could talk me through a typical day.

PATIENT: Well, I get up, have two cups of coffee, then go to work and eat a bagel for breakfast. Then, I don't eat again until the afternoon when I go home and binge.

INTERVIEWER: Can you tell me more about breakfast? When you say you had a bagel, how much?

PATIENT: What do you mean?

INTERVIEWER: Well, was it half the bagel? Three-quarters of it? Do you put anything on it or eat it plain?

PATIENT: Oh, I see what you're asking. No, it's not the whole thing. Usually half a bagel and I throw the other half out so I won't eat it. I eat it plain. And it's a low-fat bagel.

INTERVIEWER: I see. That helps me understand better. You mentioned the binges in the afternoon. Binges can mean different things to different people. Can you tell me about these episodes in more detail?

PATIENT: Well, I get home and I promise myself that I'll go exercise and I won't eat anything. But I'm usually really hungry so I'll go to the kitchen to see if my roommate has any leftover food. If she does, I'll tell myself that I shouldn't eat it, but I can't resist it so I start eating and I can't stop. Then I feel so disgusting that I'll make myself vomit.

INTERVIEWER: Yes, I understand how feeling that kind of loss of control when you're eating can be so upsetting. I'd really like to hear about these episodes in more detail. Can you tell me about one that you had recently? I'm especially interested in hearing about the specific foods you ate.

PATIENT: Well, there were leftover cookies so I ate those, and then a container of ice cream.

INTERVIEWER: Let's start with the cookies. What kind were they?

PATIENT: Chocolate chip.

INTERVIEWER: And what size were they?

PATIENT: Well, my roommate baked them. They were probably two inches wide.

INTERVIEWER: How many do you think you ate?

PATIENT: Probably 20.

INTERVIEWER: And you mentioned the container of ice cream. What size?

PATIENT: What do you mean?

INTERVIEWER: Was it a gallon? A half-gallon? A pint?

PATIENT: A pint.

INTERVIEWER: So you had the cookies and the ice cream, and what else did you eat during this episode?

This exchange illustrates the interviewer's use of detailed questioning to develop an understanding of the patient's eating pattern. For example, rather than assuming that the entire bagel had been eaten, the interviewer asked about the specific portion. In discussing binge eating, the interviewer asked detailed questions about types and amounts of food. The interviewer used subtle wording to convey a sense of acceptance of these episodes, for example, by asking if the container of ice cream had been a gallon size and asking "what else?" to imply that a consumption of large amounts of food during a binge eating episode is to be expected. Although it is important to avoid asking leading questions, the interviewer can put the patient at ease by indicating a familiarity with the amounts of food consumed during typical binge eating episodes ("So, when you said that you ate a bag of potato chips, was that a family-sized bag?").

The interviewer's words and actions will strongly affect the interview process (Turner & Hersen, 1985). The interviewer must be careful to avoid expressing subtle judgment or criticism through tone of voice and facial expressions. It is essential to display a sense of empathy and understanding regardless of what the patient says. Because diagnostic interviews are often the initial therapeutic contact, use of motivational interviewing techniques—expressing empathy, avoiding argument, and rolling with resistance—can be helpful (Miller & Rollnick, 2002).

The use of active listening skills is also an important component of interviewing, both for diagnosis and for developing a therapeutic alliance (Keel, 2001). Using summary statements and paraphrasing, that is, restating what the patient has said, serves two functions: it facilitates rapport and also allows the interviewer to ensure that the diagnostic data are accurate. Paraphrasing in the form of a question is especially effective for conveying empathy and building an alliance; however, to avoid parroting, the interviewer should not use summary statements and paraphrasing too frequently (Keel, 2001). These techniques are most useful to highlight key statements made by the patient and to clarify information that may be confusing:

> INTERVIEWER: Can you tell me about your weight patterns? How long have you been at this weight?
>
> PATIENT: I'm not really sure. About 2 years ago, I used to weigh myself constantly. Then I started to gain weight and it became so upsetting that I stopped weighing myself for over a year. I wore the same size clothes during all those months and they seemed to fit, so I don't think my weight changed. Then a month ago, I decided to change my eating patterns so I got on the scale and it was about 5 pounds heavier than what my weight is on your scale today.
>
> INTERVIEWER: So it sounds like last month your weight was about five pounds higher, and you're not really sure about your weight for the year before that but it was probably in the same range. Two years ago, your weight was lower. Is that right?

This example illustrates the use of paraphrasing what the patient has stated to convey a sense of understanding as well as to confirm the accuracy of what the interviewer has heard.

The diagnostic interviewer should expect that some patients are likely to be frightened, hostile, and ashamed. Patients with eating disorders often become tearful during interviews, particularly when discussing symptoms that cause them feelings of shame such as binge-eating episodes and negative attitudes about body shape and weight. When a patient becomes upset, the interviewer should pause briefly, make an empathetic comment (e.g., "Talking about your eating patterns seems to be upsetting you"), and assess what may help, for example, a tissue, a break, or a drink of water. For patients who find the process of diagnostic interviewing painful, the interviewer can consider conducting the evaluation in several short sessions rather than one long session. The gradual establishment of rapport usually helps to put patients at ease, and most will reveal less anxiety and hostility as the interview progresses.

In summary, developing rapport is crucial to conducting diagnostic interviewing. Rapport can be facilitated through the expression of empathy, the absence of criticism, and the use of active listening techniques and detailed questioning that indicate the interviewer's understanding of the patient's experience. Inadequate rapport can limit the accuracy of the information provided by the patient and can impede the development of a longer-term relationship and therapeutic alliance.

DIAGNOSTIC INTERVIEW INSTRUMENTS

Several clinician-based interviews have been developed to assess eating disorder symptoms and associated psychopathology. The Eating Disorder Examination (EDE; Fairburn & Cooper, 1993) and the Structured Interview for Anorexic and Bulimic Disorders (SIAB-EX; Fichter, Herpertz, Quadflieg, & Herpertz-Dahlmann, 1998) are clinician-based interviews that have been widely used in research studies of eating disorders and have reliability and validity data to support their use (Fairburn & Cooper, 1993; Fichter & Quadflieg, 2001; Rizvi, Peterson, Crow, & Agras, 2000). The Structured Clinical Interview for DSM-IV (SCID) is a semi-structured interview that can be used to assess Axis I psychopathology including eating disorders (SCID-I; First, Spitzer, Gibbon, & Williams, 2002) and Axis II personality disorders (SCID-II; First, Spitzer, Gibbon, & Williams, 1997). The EDE, SIAB-EX, SCID-I and SCID-II are discussed in detail in Chapter 5. Although these types of interviews are used primarily for research, they can also be employed in clinical settings to obtain a detailed assessment of symptoms as well as to make DSM-IV diagnoses. Using standard interviews has a number of advantages and is likely to improve the quality of data when conducting a diagnostic interview. The use of standard interviews facilitates the consistent collection of data across different settings. The structure of the interview reduces the risk that the assessor will omit important questions. Because these instruments have been piloted and modified extensively and have psychometric data to support their use, the interviewer can be confident that the questions and probes are effective in eliciting information necessary to make accurate diagnoses. Finally, when conducted skillfully, structured assessments can enhance rather than limit rapport. Potential disadvantages include training requirements, cost, and time.

ASSESSING EATING DISORDER SYMPTOMS

Introduction and Overview

Whether or not the clinician is using a structured interview, the beginning of the diagnostic interview should include questions about the patient's age, marital status and children, occupation, educational history, living situation, and, for treatment settings, referral source. It can also be helpful to ask about the patient's feelings about the interview and to ask whether there are any initial questions. The interviewer should introduce him- or herself as well as describe the purpose of the interview, the amount of time it will take, and any limitations in confidentiality.

The diagnostic interview should include questions about both current and past symptoms. Some interviewers prefer to have patients describe their symptoms in chronological order ("Why don't you begin by telling me how these problems started and talk me through what happened as things went along?"). Others prefer to focus on current symptoms and to ask about past symptoms in reference to the present ("You said that you are self-inducing vomiting twice a week. How long has this been your pattern? Do you remember how old you were when it started? Was it ever occurring more than twice a week? When was that?"). Whatever the order, for each symptom the diagnostic interviewer should identify the age of onset, current status, when it was the worst and the frequency and intensity at that time, and the course. Eating disorder symptoms to evaluate during a diagnostic interview are outlined in Table 3.1.

Eating Patterns and Dietary Restriction

The interviewer should evaluate how frequently the patient eats meals and snacks as well as their content. Although general questions can be asked about the frequency of meal consumption, the length of time between meals, and patterns of fasting, obtaining detailed examples can usually provide a more accurate picture of the patient's eating patterns. For example, the interviewer can ask the patient to describe the timing and content of food consumed on the day prior to the evaluation. Although it is not time-efficient to discuss patterns for each day in detail, it is often effective to use one example as a point of comparison with eating patterns at other times ("Was yesterday a typical day? How long has this been your typical pattern? If yesterday was unusual, how is a typical day different? Was your pattern of eating similar last month? Last year?"). Obtaining a detailed description of a typical 24-hour time period also prevents confusion that can arise from misinterpreting more general questions, for example, asking about "overeating," "dieting," "eating too little," or "restricting." However, once the interviewer has obtained objective data about the patient's pattern of eating, it is then useful to understand the patient's perspective about those eating patterns, for example, whether they are regarded as restrictive.

Evaluating dietary restriction involves both behavioral and attitudinal assessment. The interviewer should consider the three types of dieting

TABLE 3.1. Eating Disorder Symptoms Evaluated during Diagnostic Interviews

1. *Binge eating*
   a. Types of food
   b. Amounts of food
   c. Presence or absence of loss of control
   d. Length of time (e.g., time started, time stopped, breaks in eating)
   e. Different types of binge eating episodes (e.g., objective and subjective)
2. *Purging*
   a. Self-induced vomiting (include use of syrup of ipecac)
   b. Laxative misuse
   c. Enema or colonic misuse
   d. Diuretic misuse
3. *Other compensatory behaviors and associated symptoms*
   a. Fasting
   b. Exercising (including motivation, frequency, intensity)
   c. Diet pill use
   d. Chewing and spitting
   e. Rumination
   f. Smoking and caffeine use for weight control
4. *Eating patterns and dietary restriction*
   a. Frequency of meals and snacks
   b. Timing between meals and snacks
   c. Fasting and skipping meals
   d. Rules about content and timing of food consumption
   e. Avoidance of specific foods
   f. Preoccupations and rituals pertaining to food consumption and restriction
5. *Weight history*
   a. Current height and weight (obtain objective measure)
   b. Lowest past weight (and age)
   c. Highest past weight (and age)
   d. Pattern of weight fluctuation
   e. Ideal weight
6. *Body image*
   a. Body dissatisfaction (overall body and parts)
   b. Influence of weight and shape on self-evaluation
   c. Size perception and overestimation
   d. Fear of gaining weight
   e. Preoccupations, rituals, checking, and avoidance behaviors related to weight and shape

patterns typically seen in patients with eating disorders: (1) skipping meals or fasting, (2) restricting overall intake, and (3) avoiding or restricting certain types of foods (Fairburn, Marcus, & Wilson, 1993). The interviewer should establish both the frequency that these different types of behaviors occur and the accompanying attitudinal content, including rules about consuming calories, fat grams, carbohydrates, specific foods or combinations of foods, and restricting eating to certain times of day. Clinically, it can be useful to determine whether these guiding principles are rigid rules or more flexible guidelines (Fairburn & Cooper, 1993). The interviewer can emphasize to the patient that the question is about the intent to follow these rules about eating, regardless of success. Although preoccupations and rituals are not included in the diagnostic criteria for eating disorders, they often feature prominently (Sunday, Halmi, & Einhorn, 1995).

Because many patients report significant impairment due to preoccupations and rituals, this type of information can be useful for treatment planning. The interviewer can ask about the content and frequency of preoccupations, as well as the extent to which they interfere with concentration. Useful questions include asking about how many minutes in a typical hour the patient spends thinking about food and eating. The diagnostic interview can also include questions about type and frequency of rituals, especially for patients with AN ("Some people find that they need to prepare food or eat in a very specific and ritualized way, to the point that they feel quite anxious if they have to do things differently. For example, some people need to chew their food a certain number of times before swallowing or eat certain foods in a certain order. Do you have any rituals like this?"). Mazure, Halmi, Sunday, Romano, and Einhorn (1994) developed the Yale–Brown–Cornell Eating Disorder Scale (YBC) to assess rituals and preoccupations specific to eating disorders. This measure can be used during the diagnostic interview to determine content and severity of these symptoms, the extent to which they cause interference, and the patient's motivation to change them.

In summary, interviewing patients with eating disorder symptoms requires a considerable emphasis on evaluating detailed patterns of eating and food restriction. Asking the patient for specific examples of eating patterns is necessary to minimize the confusion and misinterpretations that can arise from more general questions. The focus of the diagnostic interview should include both the behavioral and attitudinal components of these eating patterns. Assessing preoccupations and rituals can also be beneficial.

Binge Eating

Binge eating is among the most difficult behaviors to assess and measure in patients with eating disorders (Peterson & Miller, 2005; Wilson, 1993). Several factors contribute to problems with assessing binge eating. First, many patients feel ashamed about these episodes. For some patients, these feelings can lead to deliberate minimization. In other patients, the intensity of their distress makes it difficult for them to remember the details of these episodes accurately. The diagnostic criteria are complicated because they require that binge eating episodes be characterized by both the consumption of "an amount of food that is definitely larger than most people would eat during a similar period of time and under similar circumstances . . . [and] a sense of lack of control" (American Psychiatric Association, 2000, p. 594).

The DSM-IV-TR criteria correspond with the binge eating classification scheme of the EDE (Fairburn & Cooper, 1993), which includes two dimensions: whether the patient experiences a sense of loss of control, and whether the amount of food consumed during the episode is definitely large. According to the EDE, an episode in which the amount of food is definitely large and the patient reports a sense of loss of control is classified as an objective bulimic episode or an objective binge eating episode. An episode in which the patient reports a sense of loss of control and believes that he or she has overeaten but the amount of food consumed is not considered large by the interviewer is considered a subjective bulimic episode or subjective binge eating episode. An episode in which the amount consumed is large, both in the opinion of the interviewer and patient, but is not accompanied by a sense of loss of control is considered an objective overeating episode. Of note, patients who binge often report having multiple types of episodes, that is, both objective and subjective (Rossiter & Agras, 1990). Although it is not usually necessary to explain this classification system to the patient, it can be extremely useful for the interviewer to understand the different types of binge eating and overeating episodes in order to assess them with greater accuracy. In fact, arguing with the patient that the amount consumed during binge eating episodes is not large is ill advised during a diagnostic interview because it communicates a sense that the interviewer does not understand the patient's perspective, which can potentially compromise rapport. However, within a therapeutic context, such interpretations can be useful if made skillfully.

Defining an amount of food consumed during a binge eating episode as definitely larger is challenging because appraisals of "large" vary by peer group, geographical location, and individual perception (Fairburn & Cooper, 1993). Perhaps the most important tool in evaluating binge eating accurately is to ask sufficiently detailed questions to yield adequate data about the amount of food consumed during these episodes. When assessing binge eating, the interviewer should ask for specific examples of binge eating episodes including types of food, amounts of food, and duration (e.g., whether it occurred within a 2-hour time period).

Many examples of binge eating are clearly large and straightforward for the interviewer to appraise. As described earlier, patients with eating disorders also report subjective binge eating episodes in which they believe they have overeaten but the amount is clearly not large to the interviewer (e.g., two small cookies). However, the interviewer may encounter examples that are more difficult to classify. Several strategies can be used. First, the interviewer can ask for additional examples, which often results in the patient describing other episodes of binge eating that are clearly large. Second, the interviewer can ask more questions about context, including what others were eating and circumstances surrounding the episode (e.g., if the episode occurred at a buffet, where overeating is more normative). Third, the interviewer can confer with colleagues to try to reach consensus about whether or not the amount consumed during the episode is definitely larger. Within research studies, it is helpful for assessors to communicate regularly with one another by meeting in person, teleconferencing, or e-mail, to discuss examples of binge sizes and establish agreement about thresholds of what is large (while taking regional differences into consideration). Finally, for cases in which a decision about whether the episode includes an amount of food that is definitely large cannot be reached, the interviewer can follow the suggestion of the EDE (Fairburn & Cooper, 1993) by being conservative and rating the episode as subjective rather than objective.

Assessing a lack or loss of control during binge eating can also be difficult. Most patients who report binge eating understand that lack of control is a subjective experience that occurs during these episodes and are able to describe this phenomenon to the interviewer. However, a minority of patients question whether they are truly "out of control" because their episodes are often planned or intentional. The probes described in the EDE are useful because they rephrase the question in more concrete terms (Fairburn & Cooper, 1993). Specifically, the interviewer can ask if the patient felt that he or she could have stopped eating or prevented the episode from occurring. If the patient responds that neither of these experiences has characterized their eating, the interviewer can infer that a sense of lack of control was present. Similarly, lack of control can be presumed if the patient reports feeling driven or compelled to eat. Once again, using specific examples can help patients understand these concepts:

INTERVIEWER: You mentioned that you are bothered by overeating episodes. Can you tell me more about these episodes?

PATIENT: Well, while I'm driving home from work I'm thinking about which restaurant to go to first. I usually pick up food from three or four fast-food restaurants, eat in the car, then stop at the gas station to make myself vomit.

INTERVIEWER: That gives me a much clearer picture. Can you tell me a little more about what types and amount of food you might eat during a typical episode? Maybe you can remember one you've had recently.

PATIENT: Well, I had one on Monday.

INTERVIEWER: Perhaps you could tell me about that one.

PATIENT: Work was terrible. Really stressful. All day I kept thinking about leaving work to go binge. By the early afternoon, I started planning where to go and what to eat. I couldn't wait for work to be over so I could leave and go binge. As usual, I drove to several restaurants. I don't want the people at the restaurants to know how much I eat so I end up buying meals at all of them. I ate as I drove and then stopped to park near the gas station to finish the rest.

INTERVIEWER: So you had a tough day at work and ended up driving to several restaurants. Can you describe more specifically what you ate?

PATIENT: Well, I remember eating two hamburgers, two chicken sandwiches, two slices of pizza, two regular orders of fries, four breadsticks, one ice cream sundae, and one piece of apple pie.

INTERVIEWER: Did you eat anything else during that episode?

PATIENT: No, that was it.

INTERVIEWER: How long did this episode last?

PATIENT: It started around five o'clock and I finished vomiting at seven o'clock.

INTERVIEWER: Were there any breaks when you stopped eating during that 2-hour time period?

PATIENT: No, I ate the whole time and then started vomiting.

INTERVIEWER: Did you feel a sense of loss of control during this episode?

PATIENT: I'm not sure what you mean. I think that I was in control because I had been planning to binge all afternoon. I knew exactly where I was going to go and what I was going to eat.

INTERVIEWER: Yes, I understand that it's a confusing question. Let me rephrase it: Did you feel like you could have stopped eating once you started?

PATIENT: What do you mean?

INTERVIEWER: Well, once you started to eat the food that you bought, could you have stopped eating it?

PATIENT: Oh, I see what you mean. Like stopping after just one hamburger? No way. I had to eat everything that was there.

INTERVIEWER: Could you have prevented yourself from having the episode?

PATIENT: No, I was completely preoccupied with doing it.

INTERVIEWER: Did you feel driven and compelled to eat during the episode?

PATIENT: Yes.

In this example, the patient did not endorse a sense of lack of control when asked initially. However, with continued probing by the interviewer, it became clear that the patient felt incapable of preventing the episode from occurring or of stopping it. The example would meet criteria for a binge eating episode in DSM-IV (and an objective bulimic episode according to the EDE criteria) because the amount of food consumed was clearly large and the episode was accompanied by a sense of loss of control.

In summary, assessing binge eating is challenging, in part, because of the complexity of determining both the size of the episode and the accompanying experience of lack of control over eating. In addition, many patients find it a difficult topic to discuss because of feelings of shame. To increase the accuracy of diagnostic assessment, the interviewer should ask for detailed examples of binge eating episodes. Rapport can be enhanced by maintaining an accepting and nonjudgmental stance during this portion of the interview as well as by using reflective listening skills and expressing empathy.

Compensatory Behaviors and Associated Symptoms

It is important to ask all patients about compensatory symptoms, whether or not they report binge eating episodes. Although objective and subjective binge eating episodes are associated with the use of compensatory behaviors in BN and AN, some patients use these methods after consuming regular meals and snacks and regardless of whether they experienced a sense of loss of control. The assessment of compensatory behaviors is typically straightforward, and patients can often remember episodes of self-induced vomiting and laxative abuse more accurately than binge eating (Peterson, Miller, Johnson-Lind, Crow, & Thuras, 2005). Current and past frequency of episodes of self-induced vomiting, including the use of syrup of ipecac, should be evaluated. The interviewer should also ask about the misuse of laxatives, enemas, and diuretics. Because patients are often confused about these terms, it is helpful to ask them to describe specifically what they are taking (including the brand name), how much they take each time, and the frequency of use. The interviewer can also ask about the intention and motivation for using these methods to confirm that the behavior is intended to prevent weight gain and influence shape and weight. For example, the use of prescription diuretics for a medical condition would not be considered compensatory unless the primary motivation was to influence shape or weight. Although less common, the following symptoms should also be evaluated during the diagnostic interview: chewing and spitting, rumination, misuse of insulin and thyroid medication, and diet pill use.

Excessive exercise is a common feature of AN and is included in the diagnostic criteria for BN as an example of a compensatory behavior. Although no clear rules define specific exercise levels as excessive, several factors should be considered. The motivation to exercise should be primarily to influence body weight, shape, or body composition, prevent weight gain, or compensate for food consumed during binge eating episodes. It can be helpful to ask the patient to list the motivations for exercise and to attempt to rank these reasons in order of importance. Several probes from the EDE are helpful to assess the psychological aspects of exercise: whether the patient feels driven or compelled to exercise; whether he or she has pushed too hard, even to the point of doing harm (e.g., exercising in spite of illness or injury); and how the patient feels when unable to exercise (Fairburn & Cooper, 1993). The interviewer can also ask about the extent to which exercise interferes with the patient's life, for example missing work or social activities. Although it is important to assess the patient's appraisal of whether the exercise is excessive and problematic, the interviewer should ask a number of detailed questions about the type, frequency, and intensity of the behaviors to make an independent decision based on clinical judgment (because some patients who engage in excessive exercise deny that it is problematic).

Weight

To make the diagnosis of AN, the interviewer must have an accurate reading of the patient's weight and height. If at all possible, the interviewer should measure weight and height at the interview with the patient wearing a gown (because some patients attempt to conceal being underweight by wearing heavy clothing and carrying weights in clothing pockets). Because being weighed is extremely stressful for many patients, this procedure should be done with sensitivity. For example, the patient should be given the choice of seeing the number on the scale or doing a blind weighing. In some clinical settings where measuring height and weight are not feasible, the patient's self-reported height and weight should be viewed as provisional until they can be confirmed by a physician's examination. Many patients are quite accurate in their self-reported height and weight. Others, however, may report inaccurate numbers for fear that revealing their actual weight during a diagnostic interview will result in hospitalization and forced treatment. For other patients, their inaccurate self-reports are unintentional.

Although the interviewer should not rely on self-reported data for height and weight, it is crucial to avoid conveying such skepticism directly to the patient. One of the most challenging aspects of conducting clinical work with eating disorder patients is to maintain realistic skepticism in the context of respect and collaboration. For example:

INTERVIEWER: Before we finish the evaluation process today, I would like to have our nurse measure your height and weight.

PATIENT: I really don't want to do that.

INTERVIEWER: Many people find it difficult. What will make it hard for you?

PATIENT: It's just too depressing.

INTERVIEWER: I'm sorry that it's something you find so painful. I really do understand how hard it can be. Are there ways that we could make it less difficult for you? For example, would you be more comfortable if you didn't have to see the weight?

PATIENT: Yes, that would probably help. Also, I hate it at the doctor's office when they yell out the number so that everybody around can hear it. I feel so humiliated.

INTERVIEWER: I understand. I'm glad you told me that. Why don't we have you turn around when you stand on the scale so you don't have to see the number. Our nurse is very careful about these things but I'll step out while you change into a gown and ask her to just write the numbers down and not say anything out loud. Would that be helpful to you?

PATIENT: Yes, thank you.

INTERVIEWER: I'll check in with you afterwards to see how you're doing.

In addition to measuring the patient's weight, the interviewer should ask about current and past weight history, including age of highest weight and lowest weight, degree of weight fluctuation, and weight patterns in childhood and adolescence. Asking about ideal weight is also helpful and can serve as a lead-in question to other aspects of body image. Similarly, the interviewer can ask about the frequency of weighing behavior and any rituals around weighing (e.g., feeling compelled to weigh at a certain time of day, stepping on and off the scale a certain number of times). Assessing the frequency of weighing is important because patients with eating disorders tend to weigh themselves quite frequently or avoid weighing altogether (Fairburn et al., 1993).

In summary, the interviewer should rely on objective measures as well as self-reported height and weight. Ideally, the underweight patient should be weighed and measured wearing a gown. Weight history should also be assessed. Because being weighed and discussing weight are both difficult for many patients with eating disorders, the interviewer should be especially sensitive during this portion of the evaluation.

Body Image, Self-Evaluation, and Attitudes about Appearance

Body image is a complex and multidimensional construct that has been plagued by assessment problems for several decades (Thompson, 2004) but is considered central to the etiology and maintenance of eating disorder symptoms (Fairburn & Garner, 1988; Stice, 2002). One of the most important considerations for the diagnostic interviewer is to recognize that there is no single method of assessing body image (Thompson, 2004), and the goal must be to evaluate different aspects of body image including perceptual and attitudinal components (see Chapter 10). The clinician must also recognize that this particular topic is especially painful for many patients to discuss and is often the most difficult component of the diagnostic interview.

Body Dissatisfaction

The interviewer should ask about satisfaction and dissatisfaction with appearance, including overall appearance, overall body shape, weight, specific body parts, and body composition (e.g., percentage body fat). Patients often emphasize that they are most dissatisfied with specific body parts rather than overall appearance (e.g., stomach, thighs, upper arms). To avoid asking leading questions, open-ended phrases tend to be most effective: "How do you feel about your body shape? What about your weight? What about different parts of your body?" The interviewer may also find it helpful to ask patients to rate their level of dissatisfaction on a 0–10 scale, and to evaluate distress, discomfort, and even self-loathing about appearance.

Self-Evaluation

Self-evaluation refers to the way in which the patient determines his or her worth as a person. The diagnostic criteria for AN and BN specify that weight and shape unduly influence self-evaluation (American Psychiatric Association, 2000). Many patients understand this concept; others find it confusing. Assessing self-evaluation can be especially challenging when interviewing individuals with limited abstract reasoning or self-awareness. In addition, some individuals find it upsetting to discussing the influence of shape and weight on self-evaluation.

In the EDE, Fairburn and Cooper (1993) provide several questions and probes to determine the role of shape and weight in self-evaluation. Patients are first asked to construct a list of the components that influence self-evaluation, and then to put these components in order. Patients can also be asked to depict their self-evaluation in the form of a pie graph (Fairburn, in press).

INTERVIEWER: I'd like to ask you a question that's a bit complicated. Does your shape or your weight influence your feelings about yourself as a person?

PATIENT: I'm not sure I understand what you mean.

INTERVIEWER: Well, let's have you start to think about a list of things that influence how you evaluate yourself as a person. This list can include things like work, school, relationships, and personal qualities. So if you had to make a list of what influences how you judge yourself as a person, what would be on the list?

PATIENT: Oh, I see what you mean. Well, let's see. I'd put my family on the list. Also, my grades at school, and what my friends think of me. My body would be on the list, too, and probably my religion.

INTERVIEWER: Excellent. Now, let's have you put them in order. Shall we write them down? That might help us get a clearer picture. Would you like to jot them down in order? *(Reaches for a blank piece of paper and pencil.)*

PATIENT: Okay *(taking the paper and pencil)*. So now I make a list of what's most important?

INTERVIEWER: Yes. But not your priorities. Those might be different. This is a list of the things that affect how you feel about yourself as a person—what would make you feel good about yourself as a person and bad about yourself as a person. Things that would influence how you evaluate or judge yourself.

PATIENT: Well, I think that grades would come first. Second would be friends and family. Is it okay that those are a tie?

INTERVIEWER: Yes that's fine.

PATIENT: Then religion. Oh, I forgot to put body on the list.

INTERVIEWER: Let's consider different aspects. Where would weight come on the list?

PATIENT: Well, honestly it's probably at the top. Although I don't know if it's more important than grades.

INTERVIEWER: Let's think about some possibilities. Which would have more influence on how you evaluate yourself as a person: a grade or a change in your weight.

PATIENT: My weight.

INTERVIEWER: And what about shape?

PATIENT: Actually, that would be the very top of the list. That would be number one, before weight and grades.

INTERVIEWER: So shape would come first, then weight, then grades.

Let me ask you to do something slightly different: What if you had to divide up a pie graph with these different pieces? So if the pie represents how you evaluate yourself and you consider your weight, shape, grades, religion, friends, and family, which would be the biggest piece of the pie?

PATIENT: Shape.

INTERVIEWER: How big would the shape piece be in the pie chart?

PATIENT: More than half.

This exchange illustrates the use of detailed questioning to determine self-evaluation. Several components of this example are notable, including the separation of weight and shape. In addition, when the patient expressed confusion about the ordering, the interviewer rephrased the question using a specific hypothetical situation (i.e., whether grades or weight change would have a greater influence). Because these cognitions are implicit, patients often do not realize how they evaluate themselves until they are asked to depict their beliefs using the list or pie graph. Ideally, the process can be collaborative as the patient and interviewer seek to understand the self-evaluation process.

Some patients deny that shape or weight are primary influences on their self-evaluation; others describe the undue influence of weight and shape in the past tense. Asking follow-up questions about how the patient would feel if weight or shape were to change can often reveal that these components have a greater influence than the patient may recognize at first. An additional question that these patients can be asked is if it is important to them that their weight and shape do not change (Fairburn & Cooper, 1993). The SIAB also evaluates this phenomenon by asking about how a 2-pound weight gain or loss would influence the patient's feelings about him- or herself (Fichter et al., 1998).

Size Estimation

The DSM-IV-TR criteria for AN include disturbance in body image (American Psychiatric Association, 2000), which typically involves overestimation of body size and shape (Cash & Deagle, 1997). Although a number of methods have been used to assess body size overestimation in research studies (Thompson & Gardner, 2002), most of these techniques are impractical to use in clinical settings. One exception is a modification of Askevold's technique (1975), in which patients are asked to use a pencil and a large piece of paper to estimate the perceived widths of different body parts.

Several strategies can be used to determine the presence of body image disturbance in the context of a diagnostic interview. First, the symptom can be inferred if an underweight individual describes his or her body or body parts as "obese." Second, some patients have an awareness of this phenomenon and will respond affirmatively if asked, "Does your perception of your body seem to shift a lot, for example, after you have just eaten?" Finally, the interviewer can ask patients directly if they believe that others perceive them as thinner than they perceive themselves.

Fear of Weight Gain

The diagnosis of AN requires that the patient report a fear of becoming fat or of gaining weight (American Psychiatric Association, 2000). Of note, some patients report a fear of becoming overweight or obese. Others deny this fear but endorse a fear of gaining weight. ("You said that you are not afraid of becoming overweight, but how would you feel if you gained five pounds? Does that possibility frighten you?") To determine the intensity of the fear, the interviewer can ask the patient to rate the intensity of the fear on a 0–10 scale.

Preoccupations, Rituals, and Checking and Avoidance Behaviors

Although not required for the diagnosis of an eating disorder, many patients report preoccupations with shape and weight (e.g., clothing size, the number on the scale) along with rituals, checking, and avoidance behaviors that are clinically significant (e.g., weighing multiple times a day, measuring body parts, scrutinizing shape in the mirror). The interviewer can ask about the frequency and intensity of thoughts about weight and shape and the extent to which these preoccupations interfere with concentration (Fairburn & Cooper, 1993). The YBC (Mazure et al., 1994) can also be used to obtain a comprehensive list of preoccupations and rituals related to shape and weight as well as to determine their severity. Asking about checking and avoidance behaviors related to shape and weight can also be useful (Cooper, Fairburn, & Hawker, 2003).

Summary

In summary, evaluating body image actually requires assessing a number of different components including dissatisfaction, self-evaluation, size perception, attitudes about gaining weight, preoccupations, rituals, and checking and avoidance behaviors. Because of the intensity of their distress about their weight and shape, patients often find these questions upsetting and the interviewer must be especially attuned to the patient's feelings during this portion of the interview. The use of concrete examples can be helpful to illustrate complex components, especially self-evaluation.

ADDITIONAL COMPONENTS OF THE DIAGNOSTIC INTERVIEW

Table 3.2 includes other topics that can be discussed during the diagnostic interview, depending on the needs of the evaluation and time available. These topics include developmental history, psychosocial functioning, medical history, and family history. If not covered sufficiently during the diagnostic interview, these topics they may be addressed during other evaluations (e.g., physical examination, psychological testing).

ASSESSING COMORBID PSYCHOPATHOLOGY

Because eating disorders are associated with high rates of comorbid psychopathology, including mood, anxiety, substance use, and personality disorders (Mitchell & Mussell, 1995; Wonderlich & Mitchell, 1997), assessing these symptoms is an important aspect of the diagnostic interview. A list of these conditions is included in Table 3.3. The interviewer can also use the SCID-I and SCID-II to evaluate these symptoms. Although a detailed description of evaluating each of these disorders is beyond the scope of this chapter, the following section includes specific considerations for assessing these comorbid conditions among patients with eating disorders.

Mood Disorders

The most critical component of assessing symptoms of a mood disorder is to evaluate current suicidal ideation and risk of self-harm. If the patient reports suicidal ideation, the interviewer should ask follow-up questions to determine if the patient has a specific plan and the current motivation to act on such a plan. It is often helpful to ask the patient if he or she is considering acting on these thoughts, as well as whether the patient has made any previous suicide attempts. Because of the high rate of depression and suicidal ideation among patients with eating disorders (Laessle,

TABLE 3.2. Additional Questions Included in the Diagnostic Interview

1. *Previous treatment*
   a. Inpatient
   b. Day treatment or partial hospital treatment
   c. Outpatient individual therapy
   d. Outpatient group therapy
   e. Medication
   f. Self-help groups
2. *Medical history*
   a. Current status
   b. Medications and allergies
   c. Menstrual history (age of onset, current and previous amenorrhea, use of birth control pills or hormones, duration of periods)
   d. Diabetes (and insulin manipulation)
   e. History of electrolyte problems
   f. GI complaints (e.g., constipation, diarrhea)
   g. Physical symptoms and pain
   h. Fainting or dizziness
   i. Dental problems
3. *Family history*
   a. Obesity
   b. Diabetes
   c. Eating disorders (bulimia nervosa, anorexia nervosa, binge eating)
   d. Mood disorders, including suicidal and self-injurious behavior
   e. Anxiety disorders
   f. Substance abuse or dependence
   g. Antisocial behaviors
   h. Psychiatric hospitalizations
4. *Social and developmental history*
   a. Childhood and adolescent family, social, and academic functioning
   b. Adult family, social, and academic and occupational functioning
   c. History of abuse
5. *Current psychosocial functioning and impairment*
   a. Relationships (marriage or dating, family, friendships, coworkers)
   b. Occupational
   c. Academic
   d. Sexual relationships (including sexual orientation)
   e. Leisure time (e.g., hobbies, activities)

TABLE 3.3. Comorbid Psychopathological Symptoms (Current and Past)

- Depression (including suicidal ideation, plan, and past suicide attempts)
- Dysthymia
- Mania and hypomania
- Substance abuse and dependence
- Panic attacks and agoraphobia
- Obsessions and compulsions (not related to eating, food, weight, shape)
- Phobias, including social anxiety
- Trauma history and posttraumatic stress disorder
- Self-injurious behaviors
- Impulse control problems (e.g., gambling, shoplifting)
- Antisocial behaviors
- Sexual dysfunction
- Psychotic symptoms
- Axis II personality disorder symptoms

Kittl, Fichter, Wittchen, & Pirke, 1987; Viesselman & Roig, 1985), all patients should be asked about current depression and suicidal ideation, including those who do not appear to be dysphoric or distressed. Patients who are not able to assure the interviewer of their safety or who appear to be at acute risk of self-injury should be accompanied to a hospital emergency room or crisis treatment setting immediately.

A consideration in diagnosing major depression among patients with eating disorders is the DSM-IV—TR criterion pertaining to changes in weight and appetite (American Psychiatric Association, 2000). For most patients with eating disorders, changes in weight are intentional and should not be counted as symptoms of depression. In a minority of cases, patients can identify eating and weight changes independent of the eating disorder that can then be counted toward the diagnosis of major depression.

Anxiety Disorders

Several issues complicate making the comorbid diagnosis of anxiety disorders among patients with eating disorders. First, patients should not be given a separate anxiety disorder if the focus of their anxiety is circumscribed to eating, weight, or shape, or any combination of these factors. For example, patients with AN who report obsessive calorie counting or compulsions related to weighing themselves or preparing food should not be given a separate diagnosis of obsessive–compulsive disorder. However, a patient who reports obsessive–compulsive symptoms with content that is not related to the eating disorder (e.g., contamination) as well as obsessions and compulsions that focus on eating and appearance can be given the diagnosis of obsessive–compulsive disorder. The interviewer may need to obtain a comprehensive list of obsessions and compulsions in order to make this determination. Similarly, patients who are afraid of eating or speaking in public primarily because of self-consciousness about weight and shape should not be given a separate diagnosis of social phobia. However, patients who describe concerns about weight and shape secondary to the public speaking itself can be given the diagnosis. Finally, because many patients with eating disorders consume large amounts of caffeine or stimulants as appetite suppressants, these substances should be ruled out as causal factors of anxiety.

Substance Use Disorders

In general, starting with open-ended questions is the most effective way of obtaining accurate data about the use of drugs and alcohol (e.g., "Tell me about your drinking habits"; First et al., 2002). Because small amounts of substances can intoxicate individuals who are underweight, the interviewer should ask specific questions about problematic behaviors (e.g., driving while intoxicated) rather than inferring problematic substance use and dependence solely by the amount consumed. For example, an individual who is severely underweight and reports having only three drinks twice each month may still meet criteria for alcohol abuse if those occasions include driving while intoxicated.

Personality Disorders

A comorbid personality disorder diagnosis should be given if the symptoms are clearly independent of Axis I symptoms, including eating disorders (First et al., 1997). However, separating personality disorder symptoms from the eating disorder can be difficult for both the patient and the interviewer, especially when the eating disorder symptoms have been chronic. Patients often have trouble differentiating problematic aspects of their personality from symptoms of their eating disorder. This process is also challenging among patients whose eating disorder symptoms are egosyntonic because their eating disorder is often perceived as part of their personality. Obtaining data from previous treatment providers and family members can be helpful in making an accurate personality disorder diagnosis.

SUMMARY

Diagnostic interviewing is a skill that facilitates an accurate assessment, which sets the stage for successful treatment. It requires that the interviewer have extensive knowledge of eating disorder symptoms as well as the clinical skills to ask difficult questions while being sensitive and empathetic. Assessing patients with eating disorders can be problematic for a number of reasons, including the limitations in the accuracy of self-report and complexity of the diagnostic symptoms. Establishing rapport during the diagnostic interview is absolutely critical. In clinical settings, rapport provides the initial foundation in building a therapeutic alliance. In both research and clinical settings, good rapport is necessary for collecting accurate diagnostic information. The diagnostic interviewer must be respectful and supportive of the patient and convey an accepting and nonjudgmental tone through both verbal and nonverbal communication.

Diagnosing eating disorders accurately requires a thorough and precise evaluation of symptoms. In assessing symptoms like binge eating, dietary restriction, and attitudes toward body shape and weight, the interviewer can ask the patient to provide specific examples in order to prevent misinterpretation. Hypothetical examples can also be provided to help with the assessment of certain psychological variables, including intense fear of weight gain and a sense of lack of control during binge eating episodes. Finally, the interviewer can potentially improve the accuracy of the diagnosis by incorporating empirically-supported assessment interviews and questionnaires as part of the evaluation process.

REFERENCES

American Psychiatric Association. (2000). *Diagnostic and statistical manual of mental disorders* (4th ed., text rev.). Washington, DC: Author.

Anderson, D. A., & Paulosky, C. A. (2004). Psychological assessment of eating disorders and related features. In J. K. Thompson (Ed.), *Handbook of eating disorders and obesity* (pp. 112–129). New York: Wiley.

Askevold, R. (1975). Measuring body image: Preliminary report on a new method. *Psychotherapeutics and Psychosomatics, 26*, 71–77.

Cash, T. F., & Deagle, E. A. (1997). The nature and extent of body-image disturbances in anorexia nervosa and bulimia nervosa: A meta-analysis. *International Journal of Eating Disorders, 22*, 107–125.

Cooper, Z., Fairburn, C. G., & Hawker, D. M. (2003). *Cognitive-behavioral treatment of obesity: A clinician's guide*. New York: Guilford Press.

Fairburn, C. G., & Cooper, Z. (1993). The Eating Disorder Examination (12th ed.).

In C. G. Fairburn & G. T. Wilson (Eds.), *Binge eating: Nature, assessment, and treatment* (pp. 317–360). New York: Guilford Press.

Fairburn, C. G., & Garner, D. M. (1988). Diagnostic criteria for anorexia nervosa and bulimia nervosa: The importance of attitudes toward shape and weight. In D. Garner & P. Garfinkel (Eds.), *Diagnostic issues in anorexia nervosa and bulimia nervosa* (pp. 36–55). New York: Brunner/Mazel.

Fairburn, C. G., Marcus, M. D., & Wilson, G. T. (1993). Cognitive-behavioral therapy for binge eating and bulimia nervosa: A comprehensive treatment manual. In C. G. Fairburn & G. T. Wilson (Eds.), *Binge eating: Nature, assessment, and treatment* (pp. 361–404). New York: Guilford Press.

Fichter, M. M., & Quadflieg, N. (2001). The Structured Interview for Anorexic and Bulimic Disorders for DSM-IV and ICD-10 (SIAB-EX): Reliability and validity. *European Psychiatry, 16*, 38–48.

Fichter, M. M., Herpertz, S., Quadflieg, N., & Herpertz-Dahlmann, B. (1998). Structured Interview for Anorexic and Bulimic Disorders for DSM-IV and ICD-10: Updated (3rd) revision. *International Journal of Eating Disorders, 24*, 227–249.

First, M. B., Spitzer, R. L., Gibbon, M., & Williams, J. B. W. (1997). *Structured Clinical Interview for DSM-IV Personality Disorders (SCID-II)*. Washington, DC: American Psychiatric Press.

First, M. B., Spitzer, R. L., Gibbon, M., & Williams, J. B. W. (2002). *Structured Clinical Interview for DSM-IV-TR Axis I Disorders—Patient Edition (SCID-I/P)*. New York: Biometrics Research, New York State Psychiatric Institute.

Keel, P. K. (2001). Basic counseling techniques. In J. E. Mitchell (Ed.), *The outpatient treatment of eating disorders: A guide for therapists, dietitians, and physicians* (pp. 119–143). Minneapolis: University of Minnesota Press.

Laessle, R. G., Kittl, S., Fichter, M. M., Wittchen, H., & Pirke, K. M. (1987). Major affective disorder in anorexia nervosa and bulimia: A descriptive diagnostic study. *British Journal of Psychiatry, 151*, 785–789.

Mazure, C. M., Halmi, K. A., Sunday, S. R., Romano, S. J., & Einhorn, A. M. (1994). Yale–Brown–Cornell Eating Disorder Scale: Development, use, reliability, and validity. *Journal of Psychiatric Research, 28*, 425–445.

Miller, W. R., & Rollnick, S. (2002). *Motivational interviewing (2nd ed.): Preparing people for change*. New York: Guilford Press.

Mitchell, J. E., & Mussell, M. P. (1995). Comorbidity and binge eating disorder. *Addictive Behaviors, 20*, 725–732.

Peterson, C. B., & Miller, K. B. (2005). Assessment of eating disorders. In S. Wonderlich, J. E. Mitchell, M. de Zwaan, & H. Steiger (Eds.), *Eating Disorders Review, Part I* (pp. 105–126). Oxford, UK: Radcliffe.

Peterson, C. B., Miller, K. B., Johnson-Lind, J., Crow, S. J., & Thuras, P. (2005). *The accuracy of symptom recall in eating disorders*. Manuscript submitted for publication.

Rizvi, S. L., Peterson, C. B., Crow, S. J., & Agras, W. S. (2000). Test–retest reliability of the Eating Disorder Examination. *International Journal of Eating Disorders, 28*, 311–316.

Rossiter, E., & Agras, W. S. (1990). An empirical test of the DSM-III-R definition of binge. *International Journal of Eating Disorders, 9*, 513–518.

Schacter, D. L. (1999). The seven sins of memory: Insights from psychology and cognitive neuroscience. *American Psychologist, 54*, 182–203.

Stice, E. (2002). Risk and maintenance factors for eating pathology: A meta-analytic review. *Psychological Bulletin, 128*, 825–848.

Sunday, S. R., Halmi, K. A., & Einhorn, A. (1995). The Yale–Brown–Cornell Eating Disorder Scale: A new scale to assess eating disorder symptomatology. *International Journal of Eating Disorders, 18*, 237–245.

Thompson, J. K. (2004). The (mis)measurement of body image: Ten strategies to improve assessment for applied and research purposes. *Body Image, 1*, 7–14.

Thompson, J. K., & Gardner, R. M. (2002). Measuring perceptual body image among adolescents and adults. In T. F. Cash & T. Pruzinsky (Eds.), *Body image: A handbook of theory, research, and clinical practice* (pp. 135–141). New York: Guilford Press.

Turner, S. M., & Hersen, M. (1985). The interviewing process. In M. Hersen & S. M. Turner (Eds.), *Diagnostic interviewing* (pp. 3–23). New York: Plenum Press.

Viesselman, J. O., & Roig, M. (1985). Depression and suicidality in eating disorders. *Journal of Clinical Psychiatry, 46*, 118–124.

Vitousek, K. B., Daly, J., & Heiser, C. (1991). Reconstructing the internal world of the eating-disordered individual: Overcoming denial and distortion in self-report. *International Journal of Eating Disorders, 10*, 647–666.

Wilson, G. T. (1993). Assessment of binge eating. In C. G. Fairburn & G. T. Wilson (Eds.), *Binge eating: Nature, assessment, and treatment* (pp. 227–249). New York: Guilford Press.

Wonderlich, S. A., & Mitchell, J. E. (1997). Eating disorders and comorbidity: Empirical, conceptual, and clinical implications. *Psychopharmacology Bulletin, 33*, 381–390.

CHAPTER 4

A Standardized Database

James E. Mitchell

As outlined elsewhere in this volume, a variety of strategies can be used to gather information during the process of the psychosocial assessment of people with eating disorders. An in-depth psychiatric or psychological evaluation obviously will be the mainstay of any assessment, as outlined in Chapter 2. As discussed, certain psychometric instruments may also provide useful data both in assessing patients before treatment and in charting their course during treatment and afterward. Other potential sources of information include interviewing family members, and obtaining prior records, particularly those related to issues surrounding mental health.

Another strategy, perhaps underutilized but nonetheless able to provide a great deal of useful information, is to use a standardized database system. An example of such a database is included in this chapter, following this introduction. Such a database can be provided to patients when they call for evaluation. They can then be asked to complete it and bring it with them to the evaluation session, to send it in advance, or to come early for the evaluation and complete it at the clinician's office. Having the patient complete it at home has several advantages in that it allows the patient to discuss questions with other family members (e.g. establishing the dates of hospitalization), to check the names and dosages of medications, and in certain situations to contact previous health care providers for additional information. While asking patients to complete such a database may seem to be assigning them an onerous task, in reality many patients see the utility of it from the beginning. First, this allows them an opportunity to organize their history in a way that they can be assured that the evaluating clinician has a relatively complete set of information about them. Second, as noted, it allows them to gather information that may not be easily recollected during the formal interview itself. Third, it assures the patient that information that cannot be covered during the interview because of time constraints still will find its way to the clinician's attention.

Clearly, the time necessary to complete such an instrument will depend greatly on the number of medical and psychological problems the patient has experienced before. Many patients with eating disorders have fairly complicated histories, and again, allowing them to complete this in advance oftentimes makes it far easier for the clinician to disentangle the time course of various problems during the interview session.

The use of such a database has obvious benefits to the clinicians as well. First, they are assured of having a reasonably complete dataset on most points of history prior to seeing the patient, allowing them to focus the interview on areas that seem unclear or that raise particular concerns; second, if the technology is available, such a database can be presented on scannable forms or via computer interface. Such technologies allow the clinician to enter the data and, if the proper software if available, print a report that summarizes the patient's responses on the items. The report so generated can become part of the permanent record. Even if neither technology is available, having such a detailed history to review immediately prior to seeing the patient can be very reassuring to clinician and patient alike.

What follows is a database that has been used in the eating disorders program in various modifications, first at the University of Minnesota and then later at the Eating Disorders Institute in Fargo, North Dakota. The version offered here is broad enough to target patients who are candidates for bariatric surgery as well as inquiring in some depth as to eating disorder behaviors such as are seen in patients with anorexia nervosa and bulimia nervosa. Given their own needs, and other sources from which they may be receiving information, clinicians who wish to set up such a database may wish to make substantial modifications to this system. Clinicians who wish to do so have permission to reproduce this instrument for their personal clinical use.

EDQ

Version 9.0

INSTRUCTIONS: Please fill in the circle that best describes you for each item.

A. DEMOGRAPHIC INFORMATION

1. Sex: O Female O Male

2. Current Age: ________ years

   Date of Birth:

   ☐☐ / ☐☐ / ☐☐☐☐

3. Race (fill in only one):
   - O White
   - O African American
   - O Native American
   - O Hispanic
   - O Asian
   - O Other (please specify) ______________________

4. Marital Status (fill in only one):
   - O Never married
   - O Married (first marriage)
   - O Divorced or widowed and presently remarried
   - O Monogamous relationship, living with partner (but not married)
   - O Monogamous relationship, not living with partner
   - O Divorced and not presently married
   - O Widowed and not presently remarried

5. What is your primary role? (fill in only one)
   - O Wage earner, full-time
   - O Wage earner, part-time
   - O Student, full-time
   - O Student, part-time
   - O Homemaker
   - O Unemployed
   - O Other (specify) ______________

B. WEIGHT HISTORY

1. Current Weight: ☐☐☐ lbs.

2. Current Height: ☐ ft. ☐☐ in.

3. I would like to weigh: ☐☐☐ lbs.

4. **Highest Weight** (non-pregnancy) since age 18:

   Weight ☐☐☐ lbs. **at** **Age** ☐☐ yrs.

5. **Lowest Weight** since age 18:

   Weight ☐☐☐ lbs. **at** **Age** ☐☐ yrs.

6. **Highest Weight between ages 12 and 18:**

   Weight ☐☐☐ lbs. **at** **Height** ☐ ft. ☐☐ in. **at age** O 12 O 13 O 14 O 15 O 16 O 17

7. **Lowest Weight between ages 12 and 18:**

   Weight ☐☐☐ lbs. **at** **Height** ☐ ft. ☐☐ in. **at age** O 12 O 13 O 14 O 15 O 16 O 17

8. At your current weight, do you feel that you are:
   - O Extremely thin
   - O Moderately thin
   - O Slightly thin
   - O Normal weight
   - O Slightly overweight
   - O Moderately overweight
   - O Extremely overweight

9. How much do you fear gaining weight?
   - O Not at all
   - O Slightly
   - O Moderately
   - O Very much
   - O Extremely

Continue on Next Page

10. How dissatisfied are you with the way your body is proportioned?

 O Not at all dissatisfied
 O Slightly dissatisfied
 O Moderately dissatisfied
 O Very dissatisfied
 O Extremely dissatisfied

11. How important is your weight and shape in affecting how you feel about yourself as a person?

 O Not at all important
 O Slightly important
 O Moderately important
 O Very important
 O Extremely important

12. How fat do you currently feel?

 O Not at all fat
 O Slightly fat
 O Fat
 O Very fat
 O Extremely fat

13. **Please indicate on the scales below how you feel about different areas of your body.** (Fill in the circle of best response for each body part.)

	(a) Face	(b) Arms	(c) Shoulders	(d) Breasts	(e) Stomach	(f) Waist	(g) Hips	(h) Buttocks	(i) Thighs
Extremely positive	O	O	O	O	O	O	O	O	O
Moderately positive	O	O	O	O	O	O	O	O	O
Slightly positive	O	O	O	O	O	O	O	O	O
Neutral	O	O	O	O	O	O	O	O	O
Slightly negative	O	O	O	O	O	O	O	O	O
Moderately negative	O	O	O	O	O	O	O	O	O
Extremely negative	O	O	O	O	O	O	O	O	O

14. On the average, how often do you weigh yourself?

 O Never
 O Less than monthly
 O Monthly
 O Several times/month
 O Weekly
 O Several times/week
 O Daily
 O 2 or 3 times/day
 O 4 or 5 times/day
 O More than 5 times/day

C. DIETING BEHAVIOR

1. On the average, how many main meals do you eat each day? [ ][ ]

2. On the average, how many snacks do you eat each day? [ ][ ]

3. On the average, how many days a week do you eat the following meals?

 Breakfast: [ ] days a week Lunch: [ ] days a week Dinner: [ ] days a week

4. Do you try to avoid certain foods in order to influence your shape or weight?

 O Yes (If Yes, what?) ____________________
 O No

5. Have you ever been on a diet, restricted your food intake, and/or reduced the amounts or types of food eaten to control your weight?

 O Yes
 O No (If No, go to section D, "BINGE EATING BEHAVIOR.")

6. At what age did you first begin to diet, restrict your food intake, and/or reduce the amount or types of food eaten to control your weight?

 [ ][ ] years old

7. At what age did you first begin to diet, restrict your food intake, and/or reduce the amount or types of food eaten to lose weight?

 [ ][ ] years old

Continue on Next Page

8. Over the last year, how often have you begun a diet that lasted for more than 3 days?

   ☐☐☐ times

9. Over the last year, how often have you begun a diet that lasted for 3 days or less?

   ☐☐☐ times

10. Indicate your preferred ways of dieting (fill in all that apply).

O Skip meals
O Completely fast for 24 hours or more
O Restrict carbohydrates
O Restrict sweets/sugar
O Reduce fats
O Reduce portion size
O Exercise more
O Reduce calories
O Other: ____________________________

11. In which of the following treatments or types of treatment for eating or weight problems have you participated?

(a) Supervised Diets:	Yes	No	If Yes, ages used	Weight at Start	Weight at End
Weight Watchers ®	O	O			
Jenny Craig ®	O	O			
Nutrasystems ®	O	O			
Optifast ®	O	O			
Procal ®	O	O			
Nutramed ®	O	O			
Liquid protein diet	O	O			
Others: ____________________	O	O			

(b) Medication for Obesity:	Yes	No	If Yes, ages used	Weight at Start	Weight at End
Phentermine	O	O			
Fenfluramine	O	O			
Xenical (Orlistat ®)	O	O			
Sibutramine (Meridia ®)	O	O			
Topiramate (Topomax ®)	O	O			
Wellbutrin (Bupropion ®)	O	O			
Over-the-counter diet pills (specify): ______________	O	O			
Other medication treatment (specify): ______________	O	O			
Human Chorionic Gonadotropin (HCG)	O	O			
Others: ____________________	O	O			

(c) Psychotherapy for Eating Problems, Weight Loss, or Weight Gain:	Yes	No	If Yes, ages used	Weight at Start	Weight at End
Behavior Modification	O	O			
Individual Psychotherapy	O	O			
Group Psychotherapy	O	O			
Hypnosis	O	O			
Others: ____________________	O	O			

(d) Psychotherapy for Eating Disorder:	Yes	No	If Yes, ages used	Weight at Start	Weight at End
Individual Cognitive Behavioral	O	O			
Group Cognitive Behavioral	O	O			
Interpersonal Psychotherapy	O	O			
Nutritional Counseling	O	O			
Others: ____________________	O	O			

Continue on Next Page

(e) Medication for Eating Problems/Weight Problems:	Yes	No	If Yes, ages used	If Yes, maximum dosage
Fluoxetine (Prozac ®)	O	O		
Desipramine (Norpramin ®)	O	O		
Paroxetine HCl (Paxil ®)	O	O		
Sertraline HCl (Zoloft ®)	O	O		
Citalopram (Celexa ®)	O	O		
Fluvoxamine (Luvox ®)	O	O		
Naltrexone (Trexan ®)	O	O		
Escitalopram (Lexapro ®)	O	O		
Quetiapine (Seroquel ®)	O	O		
Olanzapine (Zyprexa ®)	O	O		
Risperidone (Risperidol ®)	O	O		
Others: ____________	O	O		

(f) Self-help groups:	Yes	No	If Yes, ages used
Bulimia Anonymous	O	O	
Overeaters Anonymous	O	O	
Anorexics Anonymous	O	O	
Others: ____________	O	O	

(g) Surgical Procedures:	Yes	No	If Yes, at what age	Weight at Start	Weight at End
Liposuction	O	O			
Gastric bypass	O	O			
Gastric banding	O	O			
Other intestinal surgery (specify): ____________	O	O			
Gastric balloon/"bubble"	O	O			
Others: ____________	O	O			

12. Please record your major diets which resulted in a weight loss of 10 pounds or more.

	Age at time of diet	Weight at start of diet	# lbs. lost	Type of diet
(1)				
(2)				
(3)				
(4)				
(5)				
(6)				
(7)				
(8)				
(9)				
(10)				

13. Have you ever had any significant physical or emotional symptoms while attempting to lose weight or after losing weight?
   O Yes   O No

If Yes, describe your symptoms, how long they lasted, if they made you stop your weight loss program, and if they made you seek professional help.

Problem	Year	Duration (weeks)	Stopped weight loss program? **Yes**	**No**	Type of professional help, if any
			O	O	
			O	O	
			O	O	
			O	O	
			O	O	

Continue on Next Page

D. BINGE EATING BEHAVIOR

1. Have you ever had an episode of binge eating characterized by:

   (a) eating, in a discrete period of time (e.g., within any two-hour period), an amount of food that is definetely larger than most people eat in a similar period of time?
   O Yes O No

   (b) a sense of lack of control over eating during the episode (e.g., a feeling that one cannot stop eating or control what or how much one is eating)?
   O Yes O No

   If No to either a) or b), go to section E, "WEIGHT CONTROL BEHAVIOR."

2. Please indicate on the scales below how <u>characteristic</u> the following symptoms are or were of your <u>binge eating</u>.

	Never	Rarely	Sometimes	Often	Always
(a) feeling that I can't stop eating or control what or how much I eat	O	O	O	O	O
(b) eating much more rapidly than usual	O	O	O	O	O
(c) eating until I feel uncomfortably full	O	O	O	O	O
(d) eating large amounts of food when not feeling physically hungry	O	O	O	O	O
(e) eating alone because I am embarrassed by how much I am eating	O	O	O	O	O
(f) feeling disgusted with myself, depressed, or very guilty after overeating	O	O	O	O	O
(g) feeling very distressed about binge eating	O	O	O	O	O

3. How old were you when you began binge eating?

   ☐☐ years old

4. When did binge eating start to occur on a regular basis, on average at least 2 times each week?

   ☐☐ years old

5. What was your height and weight at that time?

   Weight ☐☐☐ lbs. **at** Height ☐ ft. ☐☐ in.

6. What is the total duration of time you had a problem with binge eating (whether or not you are binge eating now)?

   Days ☐☐ **Months** ☐☐ **Years** ☐☐

E. WEIGHT CONTROL BEHAVIOR

1. Have you ever self-induced vomiting after eating in order to get rid of the food eaten?
   O Yes O No (If No, go to question 8.)

2. How old were you when you induced vomiting for the first time?

   ☐☐ years old

3. How old were you when you first induced vomiting on a regular basis (on average at least two times each week)?

   ☐☐ years old

4. How long did you self-induce vomiting?

   Days ☐☐ **Months** ☐☐ **Years** ☐☐

Continue on Next Page

5. Have you ever taken syrup of ipecac to control your weight?
   O Yes O No

6. How old were you when you took ipecac for the first time?
   [|] years old

7. How long did you use Ipecac ® to control your weight?
   Days [|] **Months** [|] **Years** [|]

---

8. Have you ever used laxatives to control your weight or get rid of food?
   O Yes O No (If No, go to question 13.)

9. How old were you when you first took laxatives for weight control?
   [|] years old

10. How old were you when you first took laxatives for weight control (on a regular basis on average at least two times each week)?
    [|] years old

11. How long did you use laxatives for weight control?
    Days [|] **Months** [|] **Years** [|]

12. What type and amounts of laxatives have you used? (Indicate all types that apply and the maximum number used per day.)

			Maximum Number per Day							
	Yes	No	1	2	3	4	5	6–10	11–20	>20
Ex-Lax ®	O	O	O	O	O	O	O	O	O	O
Correctol ®	O	O	O	O	O	O	O	O	O	O
Metamucil ®	O	O	O	O	O	O	O	O	O	O
Colace ®	O	O	O	O	O	O	O	O	O	O
Dulcolax ®	O	O	O	O	O	O	O	O	O	O
Phillips Milk of Magnesia ®	O	O	O	O	O	O	O	O	O	O
Senokot ®	O	O	O	O	O	O	O	O	O	O
Perdiem ®	O	O	O	O	O	O	O	O	O	O
Fleet ®	O	O	O	O	O	O	O	O	O	O
Other (specify): ________	O	O	O	O	O	O	O	O	O	O

---

13. Have you ever used diuretics (water pills) to control your weight?
    O Yes O No (If No, go to question 18.)

14. How old were you when you first took diuretics for weight control?
    [|] years old

15. How old were you when you first took diuretics for weight control (on a regular basis, on average at least two times each week)?
    [|] years old

16. How long did you use diuretics for weight control?
    Days [|] **Months** [|] **Years** [|]

17. What type and amount of diuretics have you used? (Indicate all that apply and the maximum number used per day.)

(a) Over-the-counter Diuretics:			Maximum Number per Day										
	Yes	No	1	2	3	4	5	6	7	8	9	10	>10
Aqua-Ban ®	O	O	O	O	O	O	O	O	O	O	O	O	O
Diurex ®	O	O	O	O	O	O	O	O	O	O	O	O	O
Midol ®	O	O	O	O	O	O	O	O	O	O	O	O	O
Pamprin ®	O	O	O	O	O	O	O	O	O	O	O	O	O
Others (specify): ________	O	O	O	O	O	O	O	O	O	O	O	O	O

Continue on Next Page

(b) Prescription Diuretics:	Yes	No	1	2	3	4	5	6	7	8	9	10	>10
			Maximum Number per Day										
	O	O	O	O	O	O	O	O	O	O	O	O	O
	O	O	O	O	O	O	O	O	O	O	O	O	O

18. Have you ever used diet pills to control your weight?
    O Yes   O No (If No, please go to question 22.)

19. How old were you when you first used diet pills for weight control?

    ☐☐ years old

20. How long did you use diet pills to control your weight?

    Days ☐☐ Months ☐☐ Years ☐☐

21. What types and amounts of diet pills have you used **within the last month**? (Indicate all that apply and the maximum number per day.)

(a) Over-the-counter:	Yes	No	1	2	3	4	5	6	7	8	9	10	>10
			Maximum Number per Day										
Dexatrim®	O	O	O	O	O	O	O	O	O	O	O	O	O
Dietac®	O	O	O	O	O	O	O	O	O	O	O	O	O
Acutrim®	O	O	O	O	O	O	O	O	O	O	O	O	O
Protrim®	O	O	O	O	O	O	O	O	O	O	O	O	O
Ma Huang	O	O	O	O	O	O	O	O	O	O	O	O	O
Ephedrine	O	O	O	O	O	O	O	O	O	O	O	O	O
Chromium	O	O	O	O	O	O	O	O	O	O	O	O	O
Guarana seed	O	O	O	O	O	O	O	O	O	O	O	O	O
Garcinia Cambogia	O	O	O	O	O	O	O	O	O	O	O	O	O
Caffeine	O	O	O	O	O	O	O	O	O	O	O	O	O
Other (specify): ________	O	O	O	O	O	O	O	O	O	O	O	O	O

(b) Prescription:	Yes	No	1	2	3	4	5	6	7	8	9	10	>10
			Maximum Number per Day										
	O	O	O	O	O	O	O	O	O	O	O	O	O
	O	O	O	O	O	O	O	O	O	O	O	O	O

22. During the entire LAST MONTH, what is the average frequency that you have engaged in the following behaviors? (Please fill in one circle for each behavior.)

	Never	Once a Month or Less	Several Times a Month	Once a Week	Twice a Week	Three to Six Times a Week	Once a Day	More Than Once a Day
Binge eating (as defined on pg. 5, D.1.)	O	O	O	O	O	O	O	O
Vomiting	O	O	O	O	O	O	O	O
Laxative use to control weight	O	O	O	O	O	O	O	O
Use of diet pills	O	O	O	O	O	O	O	O
Use of diuretics	O	O	O	O	O	O	O	O
Use of enemas	O	O	O	O	O	O	O	O
Use of ipecac syrup	O	O	O	O	O	O	O	O
Exercise to control weight	O	O	O	O	O	O	O	O
Fasting (skipping meals for entire day)	O	O	O	O	O	O	O	O
Skipping meals	O	O	O	O	O	O	O	O
Eating very small meals	O	O	O	O	O	O	O	O
Eating meals low in calories and/or fat grams	O	O	O	O	O	O	O	O
Chewing and spitting out food	O	O	O	O	O	O	O	O
Rumination (vomit food into mouth, chew, and re-swallow)	O	O	O	O	O	O	O	O
Saunas to control weight	O	O	O	O	O	O	O	O
Herbal products ("fat burners")	O	O	O	O	O	O	O	O

Continue on Next Page

23. During **any one month period**, what is the HIGHEST frequency that you have engaged in the following behaviors? (Please fill in one circle for each behavior.)

	Never	Once a Month or Less	Several Times a Month	Once a Week	Twice a Week	Three to Six Times a Week	Once a Day	More Than Once a Day
Binge eating (as defined on pg. 5, D.1.)	O	O	O	O	O	O	O	O
Vomiting	O	O	O	O	O	O	O	O
Laxative use to control weight	O	O	O	O	O	O	O	O
Use of diet pills	O	O	O	O	O	O	O	O
Use of diuretics	O	O	O	O	O	O	O	O
Use of enemas	O	O	O	O	O	O	O	O
Use of ipecac syrup	O	O	O	O	O	O	O	O
Exercise to control weight	O	O	O	O	O	O	O	O
Fasting (skipping meals for entire day)	O	O	O	O	O	O	O	O
Skipping meals	O	O	O	O	O	O	O	O
Eating very small meals	O	O	O	O	O	O	O	O
Eating meals low in calories and/or fat grams	O	O	O	O	O	O	O	O
Chewing and spitting out food	O	O	O	O	O	O	O	O
Rumination (vomit food into mouth, chew, and re-swallow)	O	O	O	O	O	O	O	O
Saunas to control weight	O	O	O	O	O	O	O	O
Herbal products ("fat burners")	O	O	O	O	O	O	O	O

F. EXERCISE

1. How frequently do you exercise?

   O Not at all
   O Once per month or less
   O Several times per month
   O Once per week
   O Several times per week
   O Once per day
   O Several times a day

2. If you exercise, how long do you usually exercise each time?

   O Less than 15 minutes
   O 15–30 minutes
   O 31–60 minutes
   O 61–120 minutes
   O More than 120 minutes

3. If you exercise, please indicate the types of exercise you do (fill in all that apply).

   O Biking
   O Running
   O Swimming
   O Weight training
   O Aerobics
   O Calisthenics
   O Walking
   O In-line skating
   O Stairmaster
   O Treadmill
   O Stationary bike
   O Other: ____________________

G. MENSTRUAL HISTORY

1. Age of onset of menses: [|] years

2. Have you ever had periods of time when you stopped menstruating for three months or more (which were unrelated to pregnancy)?

   O Yes O No If Yes, number of times: [|]

3. Did weight loss ever cause irregularities of your cycle?

   O Yes O No If Yes, describe:
   ____
   ____

4. Have you menstruated during the last three months?

   O Yes O No

Continue on Next Page

5. Are you on birth control pills? O Yes O No

6. Are you on hormone replacement? O Yes O No

7. Are you post menopausal? O Yes O No

8. Please indicate when during your cycle you feel most vulnerable to binge eating. Please fill in the single best response.

O I do not binge eat during menstruation
O 11–14 days prior to menstruation
O 7–10 days prior to menstruation
O 3–6 days prior to menstruation
O 1–2 days prior to menstruation
O After menstruation onset
O No particular time

9. Do you crave particular foods (have a desire or urge to consume a specific food item or drink) for the few days prior to menstruation?

O Yes O No If Yes, what foods do you crave?

____
____

10. Do you crave particular foods (have a desire or urge to consume a specific food item or drink) during your menstruation?

O Yes O No If Yes, what foods do you crave?

____
____

11. Marriage and pregnancy:

	Yes	No	Does Not Apply
(a) Did problems with weight and/or binge eating begin before you were married?	O	O	O
(b) Did problems with weight and/or binge eating begin after you were married?	O	O	O
(c) Did problems with weight and/or binge eating begin before your first pregnancy?	O	O	O
(d) Did problems with weight and/or binge eating begin after your first pregnancy?	O	O	O

12. Do you have children?
O Yes O No (If No, skip to section H, "HISTORY OF ABUSE.")

(a) For your FIRST child, what was your...
...weight at the start of your pregnancy? ...weight at delivery? ...lowest weight in the first year after delivery?

(b) For your SECOND child, what was your...
...weight at the start of your pregnancy? ...weight at delivery? ...lowest weight in the first year after delivery?

(c) For your THIRD child, what was your...
...weight at the start of your pregnancy? ...weight at delivery? ...lowest weight in the first year after delivery?

(d) For your FOURTH child, what was your...
...weight at the start of your pregnancy? ...weight at delivery? ...lowest weight in the first year after delivery?

Continue on Next Page

H. HISTORY OF ABUSE

1. Before you were 18, did any of the following happen to you?

Yes	No	
O	O	Someone constantly criticized you and blamed you for minor things.
O	O	Someone physically beat you (hit you, slapped you, threw something at you, pushed you).
O	O	Someone threatened to hurt or kill you, or do something sexual to you.
O	O	Someone threatened to abandon or leave you.
O	O	You watched one parent physically beat (hit, slap) the other parent.
O	O	Someone from your family forced you to have sexual relations (unwanted touching, fondling, sexual kissing, sexual intercourse).
O	O	Someone outside your family forced you to have sexual relations (unwanted touching, fondling, sexual kissing, sexual intercourse).

2. After you were 18, did any of the following happen to you?

Yes	No	
O	O	Someone constantly criticized you and blamed you for minor things.
O	O	Someone physically beat you (hit you, slapped you, threw something at you, pushed you).
O	O	Someone threatened to hurt or kill you, or do something sexual to you.
O	O	Someone threatened to abandon or leave you.
O	O	You watched one parent physically beat (hit, slap) the other parent.
O	O	Someone from your family forced you to have sexual relations (unwanted touching, fondling, sexual kissing, sexual intercourse).
O	O	Someone outside your family forced you to have sexual relations (unwanted touching, fondling, sexual kissing, sexual intercourse).

I. PSYCHIATRIC HISTORY

1. Have you ever been hospitalized for psychiatric problems?

O Yes (If Yes, please complete the section below.)
O No

HOSPITAL NAME & ADDRESS (CITY, STATE)	WHAT YEAR	DIAGNOSIS (IF KNOWN) OR PROBLEMS YOU WERE HAVING	TREATMENT YOU RECEIVED	WAS THIS HELPFUL? Yes	No
				O	O
				O	O
				O	O
				O	O
				O	O

Continue on Next Page

2. Have you ever been treated out of the hospital for psychiatric problems?
   O Yes (If Yes, please complete the section below.)
   O No

YEAR(S) WHEN TREATED	DOCTOR OR THERAPIST'S NAME & ADDRESS (CITY, STATE)	DIAGNOSIS (IF KNOWN) OR PROBLEMS YOU WERE HAVING	TREATMENT YOU RECEIVED	WAS THIS HELPFUL? Yes	No
				O	O
				O	O
				O	O
				O	O
				O	O

3. Complete the following information for any of the following types of medications you are now taking or have ever taken:

		Took Previously	On Currently	Current Dosage	If taking currently, for what problem?
(a) ANTIDEPRESSANTS					
Prozac ®	(Fluoxetine)	O	O		
Zoloft ®	(Sertraline)	O	O		
Paxil ®	(Paroxetine)	O	O		
Luvox ®	(Fluvoxamine)	O	O		
Celexa ®	(Citalopram)	O	O		
Effexor ®	(Venlafaxine)	O	O		
Wellbutrin ®	(Bupropion)	O	O		
Elavil ®	(Amitriptyline)	O	O		
Tofranil ®	(Imipramine)	O	O		
Sinequan ®	(Doxepin)	O	O		
Norpramin ®	(Desipramine)	O	O		
Vivactil ®	(Protriptyline)	O	O		
Desyrel ®	(Trazodone)	O	O		
Parnate ®	(Tranylcypromine)	O	O		
Nardil ®	(Phenelzine)	O	O		
Anafranil ®	(Clomipramine)	O	O		
Remeron ®	(Mirtazapine)	O	O		
Serzone ®	(Nefazodone)	O	O		
St. John's Wort		O	O		
Lexapro ®	(Escitalopram)	O	O		

(b) MAJOR TRANQUILIZERS					
Clozaril ®	(Clozapine)	O	O		
Zyprexa ®	(Olanzapine)	O	O		
Risperdal ®	(Risperidone)	O	O		
Haldol ®	(Haloperidol)	O	O		
Navane ®	(Thiothixene)	O	O		
Trilafon ®	(Perphenazine)	O	O		
Thorazine ®	(Chlorpromazine)	O	O		
Stelazine ®	(Trifluoperazine)	O	O		
Prolixin ®	(Fluphenazine)	O	O		
Orap ®	(Pimozide)	O	O		
Moban ®	(Molindone)	O	O		
Loxitane ®	(Loxapine)	O	O		
Seroquel ®	(Quetiapine)	O	O		
Mellaril ®	(Thioridazine)	O	O		
Geodon ®	(Ziprasidone)	O	O		
Abilify ®	(Aripiprazole)	O	O		

Continue on Next Page

		Took Previously	On Currently	Current Dosage	If taking currently, for what problem?
(c) MINOR TRANQUILIZERS					
Valium ®	(Diazepam)	O	O		
Librium ®	(Chlordiazepoxide)	O	O		
Serax ®	(Oxazepam)	O	O		
Halcion ®	(Triazolam)	O	O		
Tranxene ®	(Clorazepate)	O	O		
Ambien ®	(Zolpidem)	O	O		
Klonopin ®	(Clonazepam)	O	O		
Ativan ®	(Lorazepam)	O	O		
BuSpar ®	(Buspirone)	O	O		
Dalmane ®	(Flurazepam)	O	O		
Xanax ®	(Alprazolam)	O	O		
Sonata ®	(Zaleplon)	O	O		

(d) MOOD STABILIZERS					
Lithobid ®	(Lithium)	O	O		
Depakote ®	(Sodium Valproate)	O	O		
Tegretol ®	(Carbamazepine)	O	O		
Topamax ®	(Topiramate)	O	O		
Lamictal ®	(Lamotrigine)	O	O		
OTHER:		O	O		
OTHER:		O	O		
OTHER:		O	O		
OTHER:		O	O		

J. MEDICAL HISTORY

1. Please list all medical hospitalizations:

WHEN? YEAR(S)	WHERE? (Hospital Name & City)	PROBLEM	DIAGNOSIS	TREATMENT YOU RECEIVED

2. Please list all other medical treatment you've received. (Include any significant problem, but do not include flu, colds, routine exams.)

WHEN? YEAR(S)	WHERE? (Doctor's Name & Address)	PROBLEM	DIAGNOSIS	TREATMENT YOU RECEIVED

Continue on Next Page

K. CHEMICAL USE HISTORY

1. In the last six months, how often have you taken these drugs?

	Not At All	Less Than Monthly	About Once a Month	Several Times a Month	About Once a Week	Several Times a Week	Daily	Several Times a Day
ALCOHOL	O	O	O	O	O	O	O	O
STIMULANTS (Amphetamines, Uppers, Crank, Speed)	O	O	O	O	O	O	O	O
DIET PILLS	O	O	O	O	O	O	O	O
SEDATIVES (Barbiturates, Sleeping Pills, Valium ®, Librium ®, Downers)	O	O	O	O	O	O	O	O
MARIJUANA/HASHISH	O	O	O	O	O	O	O	O
HALLUCINOGENS (LSD, Mescaline, Mushrooms, Extasy)	O	O	O	O	O	O	O	O
OPIATES (Heroin, Morphine, Opium)	O	O	O	O	O	O	O	O
COCAINE/CRACK	O	O	O	O	O	O	O	O
PCP (Angel Dust, Phencyclidine)	O	O	O	O	O	O	O	O
INHALANTS (Glue, Gasoline, etc.)	O	O	O	O	O	O	O	O
CAFFEINE PILLS (No Doz ®, Vivarin ®, etc.)	O	O	O	O	O	O	O	O
OTHER: ______	O	O	O	O	O	O	O	O
______	O	O	O	O	O	O	O	O

2. What is the most you have used any of these drugs during a one-month period (month of heaviest use)?

(Example: If you used sleeping pills about once a month many years ago, but not at all now, you would fill in the circle under "About Once a Month" on the line "Sedatives - Barbiturates...")

	Not At All	Less Than Monthly	About Once a Month	Several Times a Month	About Once a Week	Several Times a Week	Daily	Several Times a Day
ALCOHOL	O	O	O	O	O	O	O	O
STIMULANTS (Amphetamines, Uppers, Crank, Speed)	O	O	O	O	O	O	O	O
DIET PILLS	O	O	O	O	O	O	O	O
SEDATIVES (Barbiturates, Sleeping Pills, Valium ®, Librium ®, Downers)	O	O	O	O	O	O	O	O
MARIJUANA/HASHISH	O	O	O	O	O	O	O	O
HALLUCINOGENS (LSD, Mescaline, Mushrooms, Extasy)	O	O	O	O	O	O	O	O
OPIATES (Heroin, Morphine, Opium)	O	O	O	O	O	O	O	O
COCAINE/CRACK	O	O	O	O	O	O	O	O
PCP (Angel Dust, Phencyclidine)	O	O	O	O	O	O	O	O
INHALANTS (Glue, Gasoline, etc.)	O	O	O	O	O	O	O	O
CAFFEINE PILLS (No Doz ®, Vivarin ®, etc.)	O	O	O	O	O	O	O	O
OTHER: ______	O	O	O	O	O	O	O	O
______	O	O	O	O	O	O	O	O

3. Assuming all the drugs mentioned above were readily available, which would you prefer? ______

Continue on Next Page

Have you ever had any of the following problems because of your alcohol or drug use? (if Yes, please specify.)

4. Drinking and driving when unsafe?
   - O Yes......When? — O More than 6 months ago / O During the past 6 months / O Both
   - O No

5. Medical problems?
   - O Yes......When? — O More than 6 months ago / O During the past 6 months / O Both
   - O No

6. Problems at work or school?
   - O Yes......When? — O More than 6 months ago / O During the past 6 months / O Both
   - O No

7. An arrest?
   - O Yes......When? — O More than 6 months ago / O During the past 6 months / O Both
   - O No

8. Family trouble?
   - O Yes......When? — O More than 6 months ago / O During the past 6 months / O Both
   - O No

---

9. Have you ever smoked cigarettes?
   - O Yes
   - O No (If No, go to question 10.)

What was the most you ever smoked?
- O Only occasionally
- O Less than one pack per day
- O About one pack per day
- O One to two packs per day
- O About two packs per day
- O More than two packs per day

If you are smoking now, how much do you smoke?
- O Only occasionally
- O Less than one pack per day
- O About one pack per day
- O One to two packs per day
- O About two packs per day
- O More than two packs per day

---

10. Do you drink coffee?
    - O Yes
    - O No (If No, go to question 11.)

On the average, how many cups of caffeinated coffee do you drink per day?
- O Less than 1
- O 1 cup per day
- O 2 cups
- O 3 cups
- O 4 cups
- O 5 cups
- O 6–10 cups
- O More than 10 cups

On the average, how many cups of decaffeinated coffee do you drink per day?
- O Less than 1
- O 1 cup per day
- O 2 cups
- O 3 cups
- O 4 cups
- O 5 cups
- O 6–10 cups
- O More than 10 cups

---

11. Do you drink tea?
    - O Yes
    - O No (If No, go to question 12.)

On the average, how many cups of caffeinated tea do you drink per day?
- O Less than 1
- O 1 cup per day
- O 2 cups
- O 3 cups
- O 4 cups
- O 5 cups
- O 6–10 cups
- O More than 10 cups

On the average, how many cups of decaffeinated tea do you drink per day?
- O Less than 1
- O 1 cup per day
- O 2 cups
- O 3 cups
- O 4 cups
- O 5 cups
- O 6–10 cups
- O More than 10 cups

---

12. Do you drink cola or soft drinks?
    - O Yes
    - O No (If No, go to next section.)

On the average, how many cans/glasses of caffeinated cola or soft drinks do you drink per day?
- O Less than 1
- O 1 can per day
- O 2 cans
- O 3 cans
- O 4 cans
- O 5 cans
- O 6–10 cans
- O More than 10 cans

On the average, how many cans/glasses of decaffeinated cola or soft drinks do you drink per day?
- O Less than 1
- O 1 can per day
- O 2 cans
- O 3 cans
- O 4 cans
- O 5 cans
- O 6–10 cans
- O More than 10 cans

Continue on Next Page

L. FAMILY MEMBERS

1.

	NAME	AGE IF LIVING	CAUSE OF DEATH	AGE AT DEATH
FATHER				
MOTHER				
BROTHERS & SISTERS				
SPOUSE				
CHILD 1				
CHILD 2				
CHILD 3				
CHILD 4				

2. Are you a twin? O Yes O No
(If Yes, is your twin identical? ____Yes ____No)

3. Were you adopted? O Yes O No
(If Yes, at what age were you adopted? _____)

M. FAMILY MEDICAL AND PSYCHIATRIC HISTORY

1. Fill in the circle in the column of any of your *blood relatives* who has, or has had, the following conditions or problems:

** Include half brothers/half sisters*

CONDITIONS	MOTHER	FATHER	*BROTHERS	*SISTERS	UNCLES	AUNTS	GRANDPARENTS	CHILDREN
Alcoholism or Drug Abuse	O	O	O	O	O	O	O	O
Anorexia Nervosa	O	O	O	O	O	O	O	O
Anxiety	O	O	O	O	O	O	O	O
Arthritis/Rheumatism	O	O	O	O	O	O	O	O
Asthma, Hay Fever, or Allergies	O	O	O	O	O	O	O	O
Binge Eating	O	O	O	O	O	O	O	O
Birth Defects	O	O	O	O	O	O	O	O
Bleeding Problems	O	O	O	O	O	O	O	O
Bulimia Nervosa	O	O	O	O	O	O	O	O
Cataracts	O	O	O	O	O	O	O	O
Cancer or Leukemia	O	O	O	O	O	O	O	O
Colitis	O	O	O	O	O	O	O	O
Deafness	O	O	O	O	O	O	O	O
Depression	O	O	O	O	O	O	O	O
Diabetes	O	O	O	O	O	O	O	O
Drug Abuse	O	O	O	O	O	O	O	O
Epilepsy (seizures, fits)	O	O	O	O	O	O	O	O
Eczema	O	O	O	O	O	O	O	O
Gall Bladder Malfunction	O	O	O	O	O	O	O	O
Gambling	O	O	O	O	O	O	O	O
Glaucoma	O	O	O	O	O	O	O	O
Gout	O	O	O	O	O	O	O	O
Heart Attack	O	O	O	O	O	O	O	O
Heart Disease	O	O	O	O	O	O	O	O
Hyperlipidemia (excessive fat in blood)	O	O	O	O	O	O	O	O

CONDITIONS	MOTHER	FATHER	*BROTHERS	*SISTERS	UNCLES	AUNTS	GRANDPARENTS	CHILDREN
Hypertension (high blood pressure)	O	O	O	O	O	O	O	O
Jail or Prison	O	O	O	O	O	O	O	O
Kidney Disease	O	O	O	O	O	O	O	O
Liver Cirrhosis	O	O	O	O	O	O	O	O
Manic Depression (Bipolar)	O	O	O	O	O	O	O	O
Mental Retardation	O	O	O	O	O	O	O	O
Migraine or Sick Headaches	O	O	O	O	O	O	O	O
Nerve Diseases (Parkinson's, MS, etc.)	O	O	O	O	O	O	O	O
Obesity (overweight)	O	O	O	O	O	O	O	O
Psychiatric Hospitalization	O	O	O	O	O	O	O	O
Thyroid Disease/Goiter	O	O	O	O	O	O	O	O
Pernicious Anemia	O	O	O	O	O	O	O	O
Psychosis	O	O	O	O	O	O	O	O
Rheumatic Fever	O	O	O	O	O	O	O	O
Schizophrenia	O	O	O	O	O	O	O	O
Sickle Cell Disease	O	O	O	O	O	O	O	O
Stroke	O	O	O	O	O	O	O	O
Suicide Attempt	O	O	O	O	O	O	O	O
Suicide (completed)	O	O	O	O	O	O	O	O
Syphilis	O	O	O	O	O	O	O	O
Tuberculosis (TB)	O	O	O	O	O	O	O	O
Other Glandular Diseases	O	O	O	O	O	O	O	O
Ulcers	O	O	O	O	O	O	O	O
Yellow Jaundice	O	O	O	O	O	O	O	O
Other: ________________	O	O	O	O	O	O	O	O

Continue on Next Page

2. If any of your *blood relatives* have not had ANY of the above conditions or problems, please indicate here:
   O Mother O Brothers O Uncles O Grandparents
   O Father O Sisters O Aunts O Children

N. MEDICATION HISTORY

1. What medications are you now taking?

MEDICATION NAME	DOSAGE	HOW LONG HAVE YOU BEEN TAKING THIS MEDICATION?

2. What drugs, medications, or shots are you allergic to?

MEDICATION/DRUG/SHOT NAME	REACTION

O. SOCIAL HISTORY

1. Highest level achieved in school (choose one):
   O 8th grade or less
   O Some high school
   O High school graduate
   O Trade or technical school
   O Some college
   O College graduate
   O Graduate study
   O Graduate degree
   O Post-graduate degree

   Specify highest degree attained:
   O M.D./D.O.
   O Ph.D./Psy.D./Ed.D.
   O Pharm.D.
   O M.A. or M.S.
   O B.A. or B.S.
   O B.S.N.
   O Other: ______________

2. Are you now employed? O Yes O No If No, when were you last employed? ____________________

3. Current occupation or last work if now unemployed: ____

4. Were you ever in the armed services? O Yes O No
   Years of service (from when to when?) ____________________ Highest rank achieved ____________________

5. Have you ever been arrested? O Yes O No

Age(s) when arrested:	Reason(s) for arrest:	Did you spend time in jail?
____________	____________	____________
____________	____________	____________

Continue on Next Page

P. MEDICAL CHECKLIST

Fill in the circle of any of the following that you have experienced during the last four weeks. You should indicate items that are very noticeable to you and not those things that, even if present, are minor.

GENERAL:
- O Severe loss of appetite
- O Severe weakness
- O Fever
- O Chills
- O Heavy sweats
- O Heavy night sweats—bed linens wet
- O Fatigue
- O Sudden change in sleep

SKIN:
- O Itching
- O Easy bruising that represents a change in the way you normally bruise
- O Sores
- O Marked dryness
- O Hair fragile–comes out in comb
- O Hair has become fine and silky
- O Hair has become coarse and brittle

HEAD:
- O Struck on head - knocked out
- O Frequent dizziness that makes you stop your normal activity and lasts at least 5 minutes
- O Headaches that are different from those you normally have
- O Headaches that awaken you
- O Headaches with vomiting

EYES:
- O Pain in your eyes
- O Need new glasses
- O Seeing double
- O Loss of part of your vision
- O Seeing flashing lights or forms
- O Seeing halos around lights

EARS:
- O Pain in your ears
- O Ringing in your ears
- O Change in hearing
- O Room spins around you

NOSE:
- O Bleeding
- O Pain
- O Cannot breathe well
- O Unusual smells

MOUTH:
- O Toothache
- Soreness or bleeding of:
  - O Lips
  - O Tongue
  - O Gums
- O Unusual tastes
- O Hoarseness

NECK:
- O Pain
- O Cannot move well
- O Lumps
- O Difficulty swallowing
- O Pain on swallowing

NODES:
- O Swollen or tender lymph nodes (Kernals)

BREASTS:
- O Pain
- O New lumps
- O Discharge from nipples

LUNGS:
- O Pain in chest
- O Pain when you take a deep breath
- O New cough
- O Coughing up blood
- O Green, white, or yellow phlegm
- O Wheezing
- O Short of breath (sudden)
- O Wake up at night—can't catch breath
- O Unable to climb stairs

HEART:
- O Pain behind breastbone
- O Pain behind left nipple
- O Pain on left side of neck or jaw
- O Heart racing
- O Heart thumps and misses beats
- O Short of breath when walking
- O Need two or more pillows to sleep
- O Legs and ankles swelling (not with menstrual period)
- O Blue lips/fingers/toes when indoors and warm

GASTRO-INTESTINAL:
- O Have lost all desire to eat
- O Food makes me ill
- O Cannot swallow normally
- O Pain on swallowing
- O Food comes halfway up again
- O Sudden persistent heartburn
- O Pain or discomfort after eating
- O Bloating
- O Sharp, stabbing pains in side or shoulder after eating

Continue on Next Page

GENITO-URINARY:

- O Stabbing pain in back by lower ribs
- O Urinating much more frequently
- O Sudden awakening at night to urinate
- O Passing much more urine
- O Not making much urine
- O Unable to start to urinate
- O Must go to urinate quickly or afraid of losing urine
- O Pain on urination
- O Wetting yourself
- O Blood in urine
- O Pus in urine

NEUROLOGICAL:

- O Fainting
- O Fits
- O Weakness in arms or legs
- O Change in speech
- O Loss of coordination
- O Sudden periods or onset of confusion
- O Sudden changes in personality (suddenly not the same person)
- O Loss of ability to concentrate
- O Seeing things
- O Loss of touch
- O Tingling in arms or legs
- O Unable to chew properly
- O Memory loss
- O Tremulous or shaky

MALE:

- O Pain in testicles
- O Swelling of testicles
- O Swelling of scrotum

FEMALE:

- O Sudden change in periods
- O Between periods bleeding

LIST ANY OTHERS NOT MENTIONED ABOVE:

____

____

____

CHAPTER 5

Structured Instruments

Carlos M. Grilo

This chapter summarizes the use of structured instruments in the assessment of eating disorders. The past two decades have witnessed considerable growth in research attention paid to developing methods in this field. This advancement has been facilitated—much as has been true for other forms of psychiatric and personality psychopathology (Grilo, McGlashan, & Oldham, 1998)—by continued attempts at greater standardization of diagnoses (clinical entities) and development of assessment methods. The development and increased utilization of structured and standardized approaches to clinical interviewing to diagnose and characterize psychopathology during the past two decades represents a critical advance. Additional information about clinical interviewing can be found in Chapter 3.

This chapter begins with a brief overview of basic psychometric issues, which need consideration by researchers when developing, evaluating, and refining these methods, and by practitioners when deciding which instruments to incorporate into their clinical practice. Second, this chapter provides a brief overview of conceptual and clinical issues to consider when selecting and using structured instruments. The chapter then turns to its major focus, an overview of the major structured instruments for eating disorders and associated forms of psychopathology. It concludes with brief comments about future needs and fruitful avenues for clinical-research efforts.

PSYCHOMETRIC ISSUES

Diagnostic criteria and entities (diagnoses) greatly influence clinical and research priorities (Grilo, Devlin, Cachelin, & Yanovski, 1997). Attention to psychometric issues is critical for the development and refinement of measures. The quality of measures plays a central role in how quickly knowledge is obtained in any field. Detailed descriptions of basic psychometric issues are available in standard texts (Crocker & Algina, 1986; Cronbach, 1970; Nunnally, 1978; Pedhazur & Schmelkin, 1991) and specific applications to assessment methods have been well articulated (Joint Committee on Standards . . ., 1999). Briefly, structured methods must possess reliability, including internal consistency, interrater reliability, and test–retest reliability. There are no absolute rules for these reliabilities as they depend, in part, on the nature and purposes of the instrument. Validity refers the extent to which the instrument captures what it claims to measure. There are standard approaches (Crocker & Algina, 1986), yet often the basic concepts are forgotten (Malgady, Rogler, & Tryon, 1992). Basic aspects of validity most relevant to this chapter include content validity, criterion (concurrent or predictive) validity, and construct validity (structure of construct, convergent validity, and discriminant validity). As concepts increase in complexity, reliability becomes increasingly difficult to maintain. Reliability is required for validity but is certainly not sufficient for validity. These basic issues are relevant to the reader when considering different measures. These issues must remain salient to the developers of measures in order to help move the field forward.

CLINICAL ISSUES

A number of conceptual and clinical issues must be considered when choosing and using structured instruments.

Purpose

The purpose or goal of the assessment determines selection of the instrument. If the purpose is screening, a variety of self-report instruments (see Chapter 6) are likely to be indicated. If the purpose is primarily to derive diagnosis, several age-appropriate diagnostic interviews are available. If the purpose is to carefully assess the nature and severity of eating disorder psychopathology, several structured interviews can, in addition to generating diagnoses, obtain detailed information about the features of eating disorders. Last, if the purpose is to assess possible coexisting (noneating) psychopathology, several diagnostic interviews merit consideration.

Assessment Is a Process

Assessment is generally a process that interacts with the treatment or research efforts. Hence, structured assessments can generate diagnoses, provide detailed information regarding the characteristics of the problem and how it might be maintained, inform treatment planning, and measure treatment progress and outcome. Hence, the reader should consider the various structured interviews as potential fits at different stages of their clinical or research processes.

Clinical Skill

Structured interviews do not eliminate the need for clinical skill. Spitzer (1983), in a classic paper titled "Psychiatric Diagnoses: Are Clinicians Still Necessary?", noted that clinicians need to obtain and integrate considerable information necessary to make complex judgments such as diagnoses. This seminal article was the basis, along with others (Pilkonis, Heaper, Ruddy, & Serrao, 1991), for the "best-estimate" diagnosis based on the LEAD standard (i.e., "longitudinal expert all-data" from all sources in addition to the interview findings). The broader message, however, is that clinical skill is a prerequisite for effective diagnostic and clinical interviewing.

Except for a few structured diagnostic interviews developed for lay interviewers to facilitate large-scale epidemiological research, such as the Diagnostic Interview Schedule (DIS; Robins, Helzer, Croughlin, & Ratcliff, 1981; Karno, Burnam, Escobar, Hough, & Eaton, 1983) and the Composite International Diagnostic Interview (CIDI; Andrews & Peters, 1998), most structured interviews require basic research or clinical training, or both. While most developers of structured interviews indicate the need for a clinical training background and a focused training experience with their instrument to obtain "certification," some interviews—such as the Eating Disorder Examination (Fairburn & Cooper, 1993) and the Personality Disorder Examination (Loranger, 1988)—require skilled clinicians to receive particularly intensive training.

Assessment Challenges and Clinical Skill

Assessment of patients with eating disorders is challenging in many respects. An understanding and appreciation for some of these difficulties is critical. Many concepts, such as binge eating (eating unusually large amounts of food and experiencing a subjective sense of loss of control) are complex and challenging to assess (Wilson, 1993). Many patients with eating disorders have high levels of shame and embarrassment about their problem. A particularly challenging aspect of assessing eating disorders is the patient's denial or minimization (underreporting) of problems (Vitousek, Daly, & Heiser, 1991; Vandereycken & Vanderlinden, 1983). Denial is common and particularly challenging among those patients with anorexia-like presentations (Vitousek et al., 1991).

Sound clinical interviewing involving a genuine empathic (accepting) stance is widely acknowledged as a prerequisite for successful assessment. With these challenging patients, knowledgeable but gentle questioning facilitated by good structured clinical interviews can facilitate the disclosure of symptoms (Vitusek et al., 1991). Since many patients with eating disorders can be children and adolescents, clinical skill is needed to ask questions in a developmentally appropriate manner (Ricciardelli & McCabe, 2001).

Structured Interview versus Self-Report

The use of structured interviewer-administered measures to assess psychopathology and functioning has a number of important advantages. Interviewers can play an active role in the process and thus help to define or clarify concepts (and questions), which should result in greater validity. The obvious drawbacks include greater cost, burden, and unavailability of specialized interviewers. Information about self-respect instruments is available in Chapter 6.

An important issue that receives relatively little attention concerns the validity or accuracy of structured interviews versus self-report questionnaires. In most cases when discrepancies occur between methods, self-reports tend to produce higher levels of most problems than interviews (Grilo, Masheb, & Wilson, 2001a). This is frequently interpreted as suggesting the superiority of the structured interview method. However, it is not unreasonable to consider the possibility that self-report methods might remove some interpersonal barriers to disclosure (e.g., embarrassment around disclosing sensitive material). Keel, Crow, Davis, and Mitchell (2002) found that whereas agreement between self-report and face-to-face structured interview for eating symptoms was "poor to fair," the convergence was "fair to good" when the structured interviews were conducted by telephone. Keel et al. (2002) concluded that these findings raise the possibility that increased reports of eating disorder problems on self-report may be due to greater honesty, and that the two methods can be complementary. This possibility is worth bearing in mind—after all, interviews also rely on self-report. This is an area of ongoing research (de Zwaan et al., 1993; Fairburn & Beglin, 1994; Greeno, Marcus, & Wing, 1993; Grilo, Masheb, & Wilson, 2001b). Nonetheless, the advantage of experts' making ratings using established anchors has been argued forcefully (Wilson, 1993). Malgady and colleagues (1992) offer a cogent discussion of the issues of validity and the complexities of comparing lay to expert judgments.

OVERVIEW OF MAJOR STRUCTURED INSTRUMENTS

Four structured interviews specifically for eating disorders have been published. These include the Clinical Eating Disorder Rating Instrument (CEDRI; Palmer, Christie, Cordle, Davies, & Kenrick, 1987), the Eating Disorder Examination (EDE; Cooper & Fairburn, 1987), the Interview for Diagnosis of Eating Disorders (IDED; Williamson, 1990), and the Structured Interview for Anorexic and Bulimic Disorders (SIAB-EX; Fichter, Herpertz, Quadflieg, & Herpertz-Dahlmann, 1998). Three of these (EDE, IDED, and SIAB-EX) have, to varying degrees, been (1) examined psychometrically, (2) revised and updated based on research findings and changes in the diagnostic classification schemes, and (3) used in various types of clinical studies. One of them (EDE) has been adapted for use with children and adolescents (ChEDE; Bryant-Waugh, Cooper, Taylor, & Lask, 1996), and two (EDE and SIAB-EX) have been translated into different languages. Accordingly, the chapter focuses on the EDE, IDED, and SIAB-EX.

Structured interviews are also considered essential for characterizing associated problems such as other psychiatric disorders and personality disorders. Psychiatric and personality disorders are not uncommon among patients with eating disorders (Grilo, Sanislow, Shea, et al., 2003; Grilo, Sanisow, Skodol, et al., 2003) and warrant assessment for various clinical and research reasons (Grilo, 2002).

For Axis I psychiatric disorders, if using lay interviewers, the two dominant instruments from the psychiatric epidemiology literature are the DIS (Robins et al., 1981) and the CIDI (Andrews & Peters, 1998). These instruments have established reliability although there remain some questions regarding their validity (Malgady et al., 1992). For Axis I disorders, the various versions of the Structured Clinical Interview for DSM Axis I Disorders (SCID-I; Spitzer, Williams, Gibbon, & First, 1992;

First, Spitzer, Gibbon, & Williams, 1996) are the clear gold-standard structured measures for use by clinically trained interviewers. In addition, the Longitudinal Interval Follow-Up Evaluation (LIFE; Keller et al., 1987) is the clear standard for assessing the longitudinal course of psychiatric disorders. In the case of children, the Schedule for Affective Disorder and Schizophrenia for School-Age Children (K-SADS; Orvaschel & Puig-Antich, 1987) is the clear standard.

For Axis II personality disorders, the literature includes five main semistructured interviews that have reasonably comparable psychometric support (Zanarini et al., 2000). These include the Structured Clinical Interview for DSM Personality Disorders (SCID-II; First et al., 1995), the Structured Interview for the DSM-IV Personality Disorders (SIDP; Stangl, Pfohl, Zimmerman, Bowers, & Corenthal, 1985); the Diagnostic Interview for Personality Disorders (DIPD; Zanarini, Frankenburg, Chauncey, & Gunderson, 1987), the Personality Disorder Examination (PDE; Loranger, 1998), and the Personality Assessment Schedule (PAS; Tyrer, Strauss, & Cicchetti, 1983). Each of these interviews has been revised and updated to reflect changes in classification schemes. This chapter will selectively present two of these interviews (DIPD and PDE) given their current prominence in federally-funded longitudinal studies focused on personality disorders (Grilo & McGlashan, 2005).

EATING DISORDER INTERVIEWS

The EDE, IDED, and SIAB-EX each provide detailed information about eating disorder symptomatology and diagnostically-based criteria. Each of these interviews generates specific eating disorder diagnoses. The EDE provides the most sophisticated and detailed assessment of eating disorder psychology and especially about different forms of overeating behaviors. While the EDE and IDED focus solely on eating psychology, the SIAB-EX provides a wealth of information about general and familial psychopathology that has been conceptually or empirically linked to eating disorders. All require skilled clinical interviewers and specific training in the use of the instrument. A critical difference between these structured measures lies in the particularly strong emphasis on "investigator-based" judgments demanded by the EDE schedule. Specifically, it is the interviewer (not the patient) who makes final judgments about what constitutes certain behaviors (e.g., binge episodes) and how to rate severity of eating disorder features. This "investigator-based" emphasis is seen by some experts as a major advantage to the EDE (Wilson, 1993). It is important to stress that the EDE demands a collaborative interview process. The interviewer and patient should strive toward a shared understanding of the concepts and definitions.

Eating Disorder Examination

The EDE (Cooper & Fairburn, 1987; Fairburn & Cooper, 1993), a semi-structured investigator-based interview, is currently regarded as the best-established inventory for assessing eating disorders (Grilo, 1998; Wilfley, Schwartz, Spurell, & Fairburn, 2000; Wilson, 1993). This instrument has gone through numerous revisions and updated editions, and has become a primary assessment instrument in treatment studies of eating disorders (e.g., Agras, Walsh, Fairburn, Wilson, & Kraemer, 2000; Wilfley et al., 2002) as well as in descriptive studies of the psychopathology of eating disorders (Fairburn, Cooper, Doll, Norman, & O'Connor, 2000).

The EDE can generate specific eating disorder diagnoses and assesses the behavioral and attitudinal psychopathology of eating disorders. Except for the diagnostic items, which are assessed and rated for the specified duration stipulations, the EDE focuses on the 28 days preceding the assessment. The EDE assesses eating and meal patterns and the frequency of specific forms of overeating, including binge eating (i.e., consuming unusually large quantities of food coupled with subjective loss of control) for the number of binge episodes (i.e., objective bulimic episodes) and the number of days on which these occurred. The EDE assesses the specific use and frequency of different forms of inappropriate weight compensatory behaviors (vomiting, laxative use, diuretic use, diet pill misuse, and extreme restriction or fasting behaviors). The EDE also comprises four subscales: dietary restraint, eating concern, weight concern, and shape concern. Items are rated on a 7-point forced-choice format (0–6), with higher scores reflecting greater severity or frequency.

Available psychometric studies of the EDE have documented high interrater reliability (Cooper & Fairburn, 1987; Grilo, Masheb, Lozano-Blanco, & Barry, 2004; Rizvi, Peterson, Crow, & Agras, 2000; Rosen, Vara, Wendt, & Leitenberg, 1990; Wilson & Smith, 1989), adequate internal consistency (Beumont, Kopec-Schrader, Talbot, & Touyz, 1993; Cooper, Cooper, & Fairburn, 1989), good discriminative validity for discriminating patients with eating disorder from normals (Cooper et al., 1989; Wilson & Smith, 1989) and among different diagnostic categories of eating disorders (Beumont et al., 1993; Rosen et al., 1990; Wilfley et al., 2000), and sensitivity to change (Sysko, Walsh, & Fairburn, 2005).

To date, the test–retest of the EDE has been reported only twice, both times in small studies (Rizvi et al., 2000; Grilo et al., 2004). Rizvi et al. (2000) performed a short-term (2–7 days) test–retest study of the EDE in a study group of 20 women with various eating disorders. Rizvi et al. reported test–retest correlations of .70 or greater for the four EDE scales, for objective bulimic days and episodes, for vomit days and episodes, but unacceptable correlations for subjective bulimic days (.40) and episodes (.34). Grilo et al. (2004) performed a short-term (mean = 10.5 days [*SD* = 3.2, range = 6–14]) test–retest of the EDE in 18 patients with binge eating disorder (BED). Grilo et al. (2004) reported very good test–retest (Spearman) reliabilities for objective bulimic episodes (.70) and days (.71) and good (significant) reliabilities for the EDE subscales, although they were somewhat variable, with correlations ranging from .50 (Shape Concern) to .88 (Restraint). These findings suggest that—even with a restricted range (all participants above threshold for diagnosis)—persons with BED report reasonably consistent responses about binge eating and associated attitudes when administered the EDE on two separate occasions roughly (on average) 10 days apart. Thus, the EDE demonstrates good test–retest reliability for making fine-grained distinctions (e.g., rank ordering) amongst patients with BED. An unpublished study (Lozano, Elder, & Grilo, 2004) reported good interrater and test–retest reliabilities for the Spanish language version of the EDE.

Despite its widespread use, the EDE has undergone relatively limited investigation of various aspects of its validity. This is not unlike the case for other structured interviews for psychiatric problems, given the complexity of designing true validity studies (Malgady et al., 1992) and the obvious lack of a clear external validator or biological marker (Wilson, 1993). Nonetheless, to date, only one factor-analytic study (to test one specific aspect of construct validity) has been reported (Mannucci et al., 1997), and this raised questions about the structure of the measure. Two available studies (Rosen et al., 1990; Loeb, Pike, Walsh, & Wilson, 1994) have reported modest concurrent validity for the EDE items pertaining to eating behaviors as tested against prospective self-monitoring records. These studies highlight the need for further psychometric evaluations of the EDE.

The EDE has been adapted for use with children and adolescents (Bryant-Waugh et al., 1996) and this version (the ChEDE) has begun to receive research attention (Tanofsky-Kraff et al., 2003; Decaluwe & Braet, 2004). This represents a potentially important development and clearly warrants continued attention. Interviewing and assessing children is complex and requires sensitivity in addition to wording that is understandable to children (see Ricciardelli & McCabe, 2001). Findings that self-report and structured interview methods are more divergent for children and adolescents (Tanofsky-Kraff et al., 2003; Decaluwe & Braet, 2004; Passi, Bryson, & Lock, 2003) than typically observed for adults (e.g., Fairburn & Beglin, 1994; Grilo et al., 2001a, 2001b) might suggest the particular importance of structured interviews when working with younger persons.

Interview for Diagnosis of Eating Disorders

The Interview for Diagnosis of Eating Disorders–IV (Kutlesic, Williamson, Gleeves, Barbin, & Murphy-Eberenz, 1998), the fourth revision of the IDED (Williamson, 1990), is a semistructured interview designed for the purpose of differential diagnosis of DSM-IV (American Psychiatric Association, 1994) eating disorders (anorexia nervosa [AN], bulimia nervosa [BN], eating disorder not otherwise specified [EDNOS], and BED). The IDED-IV differs from the EDE in several ways. The IDED-IV symptom ratings relate directly to DSM-IV diagnostic criteria and the queries enable the interview to establish the presence or absence of all of the specific criteria. The IDED, given its primary goal of differential diagnosis, does not focus on obtaining frequency and severity data for the wide range of eating disorder psychopathology captured by the EDE. It is important to emphasize, however, that the ratings produce data that allow for sophisticated analyses of psychopathology (Williamson et al., 2002) in addition to providing diagnoses.

In a particularly impressive paper, Kutlesic et al. (1998) detail four specific integrated studies following established guidelines for psychometric evaluation of measures. These studies revealed good internal consistency for symptom data specific to diagnoses, evidence for content validity, evidence for concurrent and discriminant validity, and excellent interrater reliability for differential diagnosis of specific eating disorder categories.

Structured Interview for Anorexic and Bulimic Syndromes for DSM-IV and ICD-10

The SIAB-EX (Fichter et al., 1998) has undergone several revisions following ongoing research and changes in the classification schemes (Fichter & Quadflieg, 2000; Fichter & Quadflieg, 2001). The current version, the SIAB-EX (Fichter & Quadflieg, 2000), generates data and diagnoses consistent with both the DSM-IV and the ICD-10 schemes. The SIAB-EX assesses specific criteria for AN and BN (including subtypes) as specified in the DSM-IV and the ICD-10 schemes. The data can also be used, following an established algorithm, to generate the BED research diagnosis (DSM-IV) and various eating disorder syndromes not described in the DSM-IV. The SIAB-EX provides the interviewer with clear, specific definitions of all symptoms and criteria. Examples are provided in relation to anchor points for coding. In addition, the SIAB-EX obtains information about non-eating disorder functioning, including psychopathology (depression, anxiety, substance use) and interpersonal areas. The SIAB-EX is available in English, German, and Spanish languages. In addition, the authors have developed a self-report version and have documented impressive convergence with the expert interview method (Fichter & Quadflieg, 2000). The SIAB-EX is currently the primary structured eating disorder interview in the Price Foundation Collaborative Group multisite international studies of genetic factors in eating disorders (Keel et al., 2004).

The SIAB-EX (like its earlier versions) has demonstrated good internal consistency, a consistent factor structure across several versions, good interrater reliability, and good convergent and discriminative construct validity (Fichter & Quadflieg, 2000; Fichter & Quadflieg, 2001; Fichter et al., 1998). The SIAB manual details areas of convergence and divergence with the EDE (German translation) in a study conducted with 80 inpatients with eating disorders (Fichter & Quadflieg, 2001). Overall, the SIAB-EX and the EDE produced similar general findings, although there were numerous areas of divergences between the two instruments (Fichter & Quadflieg, 2001), some of which are attributable solely to the differences in time frames and differing criteria (i.e., the SIAB-EX follows the DSM-IV and ICD-10 systems rather closely). It is, of course, difficult to interpret divergent findings from structured interviews administered by expert clinicians. For context, it is worth noting that for personality disorders, one study found that two different well-established structured interviews (SCID-II and PDE) administered independently only 1 week apart by expert research-clinicians also produced divergent findings (Oldham et al., 1992).

AXIS I PSYCHIATRIC AND AXIS II PERSONALITY DISORDER INTERVIEWS

Structured Clinical Interview for DSM-IV Axis I Disorders

The SCID-I (First et al., 1996) is the most widely used and established diagnostic interview to assess current and lifetime Axis I psychiatric disorders. The SCID is continually updated to reflect classification changes and the authors have comprehensive training materials and consultative services. Noteworthy here is that the SCID assesses for each of the DSM-IV eating disorder categories (including BED) along with all other Axis I disorders. Age of onset is also determined for each diagnosis. The SCID has extensive published data regarding reliability. For example, in a recent interrater reliability multisite study independent from the SCID-I developers, Zanarini et al. (2000) reported kappa coefficients for Axis I psychiatric diagnoses ranging from .57 to 1.0.

Longitudinal Interval Follow-Up Evaluation

LIFE (Keller et al., 1987) is a semi-structured interview rating system for assessing the longitudinal course of mental disorders. It also assesses the nature and quantity of all forms of treatment received. The LIFE (or a modified LIFE-EAT) has served as the primary measure of major longitudinal studies of eating disorders (Grilo, Sanislow, et al., 2003; Herzog et al., 1999; Strober, Freeman, & Morrell, 1997) and of major Axis I psychiatric disorders, including depressive (Grilo, Sanislow, Shea, et al., 2005; Keller, Lavori, Lewis, & Klerman, 1983; Keller et al., 1992; Solomon et al., 1997) and anxiety (Warshaw, Keller, & Stout, 1994) disorders. Good to excellent reliability has been reported for the LIFE (Warshaw, Dyck, Allsworth, Stout, & Keller, 2001).

The LIFE measures the presence and severity of psychopathology on a weekly basis. In the LIFE, the severity of psychopathology is quantified on weekly "psychiatric status ratings" (PSRs), which are made for each Axis I disorder present. For specific disorders, PSRs are based on the following 6-point scale

PSR = 1 signifies no symptoms.
PSR = 2 corresponds to one or two symptoms of mild degree with no impairment in functioning.
PSR = 3 corresponds to moderate symptoms but considerably less than meeting full criteria for diagnosis with up to moderate impairment in functioning.
PSR = 4 corresponds to marked symptoms but not meeting full criteria for diagnosis with major impairment in functioning.
PSR = 5 corresponds to symptoms meeting full criteria for disorder.
PSR = 6 corresponds to full disorder criteria plus psychosis or extreme impairment in functioning.

Remission from disorders is generally operationalized following the NIMH-CDS (Keller, Shapiro, Lavori, & Wolfe, 1982) convention for depression as 8 consecutive weeks with PSR ratings no higher than 2 (reflecting minimal or no symptoms).

The LIFE also assesses mental health treatment utilization by obtaining detailed ratings of pharmacological and psychosocial treatments for all mental health contacts, frequency of sessions, length of treatment, and number of days of inpatient and partial hospitalization. Medication usage and dosing can be recorded on a weekly basis.

The data generated by the LIFE are well suited to life table survival methods (Kalbfleisch & Prentice, 1980). Keller et al. (1982) cogently presented the specific strengths of life table analyses (over cross-sectional methods), including—but not limited to—the ability to consider the length of illness (and time to remission). These methods, employed in longitudinal studies of eating disorders (Herzog et al., 1999; Grilo, Sanislow, et al., 2003; Strober et al., 1997) allow for sophisticated examination of the timing of changes in clinical status. The EDE assessment methodology employed by Fairburn et al. (2000) in a different longitudinal effort, although strong in that it provides exquisitely detailed information, relies on a cross-sectional ("dipstick") method, and thus no information is available on periods between the assessments conducted at 15-month intervals.

Diagnostic Interview for DSM-IV Personality Disorders

DIPD-IV (Zanarini, Frankenburg, Sickel, & Yong, 1996) is the DSM-IV version of the DIPD (Zanarini et al., 1987). The DIPD-IV is a semi-structured diagnostic interview for the assessment of DSM-IV Axis II personality disorder. Each of the criteria for all DSM-IV personality disorder diagnoses is assessed with one or more questions, which are then rated on a 3-point scale (0 = not present; 1 = present but of uncertain clinical significance; 2 = present and clinically significant). The DIPD-IV requires that criteria be pervasive for at least 2 years, and that they be characteristic of most of a person's adult life, in order to be counted toward a diagnosis. The DIPD-IV is currently the primary personality disorder instrument in several NIH-funded studies of personality disorders (Grilo, Shea, Sanislow, et al., 2004; see also Grilo & McGlashan, 2005). Zanarini et al. (2000) reported interrater reliability kappa coefficients for all the personality disorder diagnoses that ranged from .58 to 1.0 and test–retest reliability kappas (based on two direct interviews of 52 participants performed 7 to 10 days apart with the second interview blind to the first interview) ranging from .69 (borderline personality disorder) to .74 (obsessive–compulsive personality disorder).

Two aspects of the DIPD-IV are noteworthy. First, good psychometric data have been reported for the Spanish Language version (S-DIPD-IV; Grilo, Anez, & McGlashan, 2003). Second, a follow-along version of the DIPD-IV has been developed that utilizes the structure and rationale of the LIFE. This follow-along version has been used in longitudinal studies (Grilo, Shea, Sanislow, et al., 2004).

Personality Disorder Examination

The PDE (Loranger, 1988) and the revision for an international multisite trial—the I-PDE (Loranger et al., 1994)—is a semistructured diagnostic interview that assesses the presence of all recognized DSM-based personality disorders. The I-PDE contains scoring algorithms to generate ICD-10-based diagnoses. This instrument also produces dimensional scores for each personality disorder construct. This instrument specifies, for adults, that traits must be pervasive and determined to be persistent for a minimum of 5 years. In studies with adolescents (Grilo, McGlashan, Quinlan, Walker, Greenfeld, & Edell, 1998), a trait may be considered present if it is judged to be pervasive and has persisted for at least 3 years.

SUMMARY

The development and increased use of structured and standardized approaches to clinical interviewing to diagnose and characterize psychopathology during the past two decades has played a central role in the development of the field. Continued and increased attention to psychometric issues and the improvement of structured assessment methods is essential for continued advancements. It is a dynamic process. Improved characterization should enhance our models of psychopathology and our approaches to treatment. In turn, advances in understanding the core features of eating disorders (e.g., Keel et al., 2004; Williamson, Gleaves, & Stewart, 2005) could guide development and refinement of assessments.

REFERENCES

Agras, W. S., Walsh, B. T., Fairburn, C. G., Wilson, G. T., & Kraemer, H. C. (2000). A multicenter comparison of cognitive behavioral therapy and interpersonal psychotherapy for bulimia nervosa. *Archives of General Psychiatry, 57*, 459–466.

American Psychiatric Association. (1994). *Diagnostic and statistical manual of mental disorders* (4th ed.). Washington, DC: Author.

Andrews, G., & Peters, L. (1998). The psychometric properties of the Composite International Diagnostic Interview. *Social Psychiatry and Psychiatric Epidemiology, 33*, 80–88.

Beumont, P. J. V., Kopec-Schrader, E. M., Talbot, P., & Touyz, S. W. (1993). Measuring the specific psychopathology of eating disorder patients. *Australian and New Zealand Journal of Psychiatry, 27*, 506–511.

Bryant-Waugh, R. J., Cooper, P. J., Taylor, C. L., & Lask, B. D. (1996). The use of the Eating Disorder Examination with children: A pilot study. *International Journal of Eating Disorders, 19*, 391–397.

Cooper, Z., & Fairburn, C. G. (1987). The Eating Disorder Examination: A semi-structured interview for the assessment of the specific psychopathology of eating disorders. *International Journal of Eating Disorders, 6*, 1–8.

Cooper, Z., Cooper, P., & Fairburn, C. G. (1989). The validity of the Eating Disorder Examination and its subscales. *British Journal of Psychiatry, 154*, 807–812.

Crocker, L., & Algina, J. (1986). *Introduction to classical and modern test theory.* Forth Worth, TX: Harcourt, Brace, & Jovanovich.

Cronbach, L. J. (1970). *Essentials of psychological testing.* New York: Harper & Row.

de Zwaan, M., Mitchell, J. E., Specker, S. M., Pyle, R. L., Mussell, M. P., & Seim, H. C. (1993). Diagnosing binge eating disorder: Level of agreement between self-report and expert-rating. *International Journal of Eating Disorders, 14*, 289–295.

Decaluwe, V., & Braet, C. (2004). Assessment of eating disorder psychopathology in obese children and adolescents: Interview versus self-report questionnaire. *Behaviour Research and Therapy, 42*, 799–811.

Fairburn, C. G., & Beglin, S. J. (1994). Assessment of eating disorders: Interview or self-report questionnaire? *International Journal of Eating Disorders, 16*, 363–370.

Fairburn, C. G., & Cooper, Z. (1993). The Eating Disorder Examination (12th ed.). In C. G. Fairburn & G. T. Wilson (Eds.), *Binge eating: Nature, assessment, and treatment* (pp. 317–360). New York: Guilford Press.

Fairburn, C. G., Cooper, Z., Doll, H. A., Norman, P., & O'Connor, M. (2000). The natural course of bulimia nervosa and binge eating disorder in young women. *Archives of General Psychiatry, 57*, 659–665.

Fichter, M. M., & Quadflieg, N. (2000). Comparing self- and expert rating: A self-report screening version (SIAB-S) of the Structured Interview for Anorexic and Bulimic Syndromes for DSM-IV and ICD-10 (SIAB-EX). *European Archives of Psychiatry and Clinical Neuroscience, 250*, 175–185.

Fichter, M. M., & Quadflieg, N. (2001). The Structured Interview for Anorexic and Bulimic Disorders for DSM-IV and ICD-10 (SIAB-EX): Reliability and validity. *European Psychiatry, 16*, 38–48.

Fichter, M. M., Herpertz, S., Quadflieg, N., & Herpertz-Dahlmann, B. (1998). Structured Interview for Anorexic and Bulimic Disorders for DSM-IV and ICD-10: Updated (3rd) revision. *International Journal of Eating Disorders, 24*, 227–249.

First, M. B., Spitzer, R. L., Gibbon, M., & Williams, J. B. W. (1996). *Structured Clinical Interview for DSM-IV Axis I Disorders—Patient Version (SCID-I, Version 2.0).* New York: New York State Psychiatric Institute.

First, M. B., Spitzer, R. L., Gibbon, M., Williams, J. B. W., Davies, M., Borus, J., et al. (1995). The Structured Clinical Interview for DSM-III-R Personality Disorders (SCID-II): Part II. Multisite test–retest reliability study. *Journal of Personality Disorders, 9*, 92–104.

Greeno, C. G., Marcus, M. D., & Wing, R. R. (1993). Diagnosis of binge eating disorder: Discrepancies between questionnaire and clinical interview. *International Journal of Eating Disorders, 17*, 153–160.

Grilo, C. M. (1998). The assessment and treatment of binge eating disorder. *Journal of Practical Psychiatry and Behavioral Health, 4*, 191–201.

Grilo, C. M. (2002). Recent research of relationships among eating disorders and personality disorders. *Current Psychiatry Reports, 4*, 18–24.

Grilo, C. M., Anez, L. M., & McGlashan, T. H. (2003). The Spanish-Language Version of the Diagnostic Interview for DSM-IV Personality Disorders: Development and initial psychometric evaluation of diagnoses and criteria. *Comprehensive Psychiatry, 44*, 154–161.

Grilo, C. M., Devlin, M. J., Cachelin, F. M., & Yanovski, S. Z. (1997). Report of the National Institutes of Health workshop on the development of research priorities in eating disorders. *Psychopharmacology Bulletin, 33*, 321–333.

Grilo, C. M., Masheb, R. M., Lozano-Blanco, C., & Barry, D. T. (2004). Reliability of the Eating Disorder Examination in patients with binge eating disorder. *International Journal of Eating Disorders, 35*, 80–85.

Grilo, C. M., Masheb, R. M., & Wilson, G. T. (2001a). A comparison of different methods for assessing the features of eating disorders in patients with binge eating disorder. *Journal of Consulting and Clinical Psychology, 69*, 317–322.

Grilo, C. M., Masheb, R. M., & Wilson, G. T. (2001b). Different methods for assessing the features of eating disorders in patients with binge eating disorder: A replication. *Obesity Research, 9*, 418–422.

Grilo, C. M., & McGlashan, T. H. (2005). Course and outcome of personality disorders. In J. M. Oldham, A. E. Skodol, & D. S. Bender (Eds.), *American Psychiatric Association textbook of personality disorders* (pp. 103–115). Washington, DC: American Psychiatric Publishing.

Grilo, C. M., McGlashan, T. H., & Oldham, J. M. (1998). Course and stability of personality disorders. *Journal of Practical Psychiatry and Behavioral Health, 4*, 61–75.

Grilo, C. M., McGlashan, T. H., Quinlan, D. M., Walker, M. L., Greenfeld, D., & Edell, W. S. (1998). Frequency of personality disorders in two age cohorts of psychiatric inpatients. *American Journal of Psychiatry, 155*, 140–142.

Grilo, C. M., Sanislow, C. A., Shea, M. T., Skodol, A. E., Stout, R. L., Pagano, M. E., et al. (2003). The natural course of bulimia nervosa and eating disorder not otherwise specified is not influenced by personality disorders. *International Journal of Eating Disorders, 34*, 319–330.

Grilo, C. M., Sanislow, C. A., Shea, M. T., Skodol, A. E., Stout, R. L., Gunderson, J. G., et al. (2005). Two-year prospective naturalistic study of remission from major depressive disorder as a function of personality disorder comorbidity. *Journal of Consulting and Clinical Psychology, 73*, 78–85.

Grilo, C. M., Sanislow, C. A., Skodol, A. E., Gunderson, J. G., Stout, R. L., Shea, M. T., et al. (2003). Do eating disorders co-occur with personality disorders?: Comparison groups matter. *International Journal of Eating Disorders, 33*, 155–164.

Grilo, C. M., Shea, M. T., Sanislow, C. A., Skodol, A. E., Gunderson, J. G., Stout, R. L., et al. (2004). Two-year stability and change in schizotypal, borderline, avoidant, and obsessive–compulsive personality disorders. *Journal of Consulting and Clinical Psychology, 72*, 767–775.

Herzog, D. B., Dorer, D. J., Keel, P. K., Selwyn, S. E., Ekeblad, E. R., Flores, A. T., et al. (1999). Recovery and relapse in anorexia and bulimia nervosa: A 7.5-year follow-up study. *Journal of the American Academy of Child and Adolescent Psychiatry, 38*(7), 829–837.

Joint Committee on Standards for Educational and Psychological Testing of the American Educational Research Association, American Psychological Association, and National Council on Measurement in Education (1999). *Standards for educational and psychological testing.* Washington, DC: American Educational Research Association.

Kalbfleisch, J. D., & Prentice, R. L. (1980). *The statistical analysis of failure time data.* New York: Wiley.

Karno, M., Burnam, A., Escobar, J. I., Hough, R. L., & Eaton, W. W. (1983). Development of the Spanish-language version of the National Institute of Mental Health Diagnostic Interview Schedule. *Archives of General Psychiatry, 40,* 1183–1188.

Keel, P. K., Crow, S., Davis, T. L., & Mitchell, J. E. (2002). Assessment of eating disorders: Comparison of interview and questionnaire data from a long-term follow-up study of bulimia nervosa. *Journal of Psychosomatic Research, 53,* 1043–1047.

Keel, P. K., Fichter, M., Quadflieg, N., Bulik, C. M., Baxter, M. G., Thornton, L., et al. (2004). Application of a latent class analysis to empirically define eating disorder phenotypes. *Archives of General Psychiatry, 61,* 192–200.

Keller, M. B., Lavori, P. W., Friedman, B., Nielson, E., Endicott, J., McDonald-Scott, P., et al. (1987). The Longitudinal Interval Follow-up Evaluation: A comprehensive method for assessing outcome in prospective longitudinal studies. *Archives of General Psychiatry, 44,* 540–548.

Keller, M. B., Lavori, P. W., Lewis, C. E., & Klerman, G. L. (1983). Predictors of relapse in major depressive disorder. *Journal of the American Medical Association, 250,* 3299–3304.

Keller, M. B., Lavori, P. W., Mueller, T. I., Endicott, J., Coryell, W., Hirschfeld, R. M. A., et al. (1992). Time to recovery, chronicity, and levels of psychopathology in major depression: A 5-year prospective follow-up of 431 subjects. *Archives of General Psychiatry, 49,* 809–816.

Keller, M. B., Shapiro, R. W., Lavori, P. W., & Wolfe, N. (1982). Recovery in major depressive disorder: Analysis with the life table and regression models. *Archives of General Psychiatry, 39,* 905–910.

Kutlesic, V., Williamson, D. A., Gleaves, D. H., Barbin, J. M., & Murphy-Eberenz, K. P. (1998). The Interview for the Diagnosis of Eating Disorders–IV: Application to DSM-IV diagnostic criteria. *Psychological Assessment, 10,* 41–48.

Loeb, K. L., Pike, K. M., Walsh, B. T., & Wilson, G. T. (1994). Assessment of diagnostic features of bulimia nervosa: Interview versus self-report format. *International Journal of Eating Disorders, 16,* 75–81.

Loranger, A. W. (1988). *Personality disorder examination.* Yonkers, NY: DV Communications.

Loranger, A. W., Satorius, N., Andreoli, A., Berger, P., Buchheim, P., Channabasavanna, S. M., et al. (1994). The International Personality Disorder Examination: The World Health Organization/Alcohol, Drug abuse, and Mental Health Administration International Pilot Study of Personality Disorders. *Archives of General Psychiatry, 51*, 215–224.

Lozano, C., Elder, K. A., & Grilo, C. M. (2004, October). The Spanish Language Version of the Eating Disorder Examination Interview: Development and initial psychometric evaluation. Paper presented at the 2004 Critical Research Issues in Latino Mental Health Conference, San Antonio, TX.

Malgady, R. G., Rogler, L. H., & Tryon, W. W. (1992). Issues of validity in the diagnostic interview schedule. *Journal of Psychiatric Research, 26*, 59–67.

Mannucci, E., Ricca, V., Di Bernardo, M., Moretti, S., Cabras, P. L., & Rotella, C. M. (1997). Psychometric properties of EDE 12.0D in obese adult patients without binge eating disorder. *Eating and Weight Disorders, 2*, 144–149.

Nunnally, J. C. (1978). *Psychometric theory* (2nd ed.). New York: McGraw-Hill.

Oldham, J. M., Skodol, A. E., Kellman, H. D., Hyler, S. E., Rosnick, L., & Davies, M. (1992). Diagnosis of DSM-III-R personality disorders by two structured interviews: Patterns of comorbidity. *American Journal of Psychiatry, 149*, 213–220.

Orvaschel, H., & Puig-Antich, J. (1987). *Schedule for Affective Disorder and Schizophrenia for School-Age Children* (version 4). Pittsburgh: Western Psychiatric Institute and Clinic.

Palmer, R., Christie, M., Cordle, C., Davies, D., & Kenrick, J. (1987). The Clinical Eating Disorder Rating Instrument (CEDRI): A preliminary description. *International Journal of Eating Disorders*, 6, 9–16.

Passi, V. A., Bryson, S. W., & Lock, J. (2003). Assessment of eating disorders in adolescents with anorexia nervosa: Self-report questionnaire versus interview. *International Journal of Eating Disorders, 33*, 45–54.

Pedhazur, E. J., & Schmelkin, L. P. (1991). *Measurement, design, and analysis: An integrated approach*. Hillsdale, NJ: Erlbaum.

Pilkonis, P. A., Heaper, C. L., Ruddy, J., & Serrao, P. (1991). Validity in the diagnosis of personality disorders: The use of the LEAD standard. *Psychological Assessment, 3*, 46–54.

Ricciardelli, L. A., & McCabe, M. P. (2001). Children's body image concerns and eating disturbance: A review of the literature. *Clinical Psychology Review, 21*, 325–344.

Rizvi, S. L., Peterson, C. B., Crow, S. J., & Agras, W. S. (2000). Test–retest reliability of the Eating Disorder Examination. *International Journal of Eating Disorders, 28*, 311–316.

Robins, L. N., Helzer, J. E., Croughlin, J., & Ratcliff, K. S. (1981). National Institute of Mental Health Diagnostic Interview Schedule: Its history, characteristics, and validity. *Archives of General Psychiatry, 38*, 381–389.

Rosen, J. C., Vara, L., Wendt, S., & Leitenberg, H. (1990). Validity studies of the Eating Disorder Examination. *International Journal of Eating Disorders, 9*, 519–528.

Solomon, D. A., Keller, M. B., Leon, A. C., Mueller, T. I., Shea, M. T., Warshaw, M., et al. (1997). Recovery from major depression: A 10-year prospective follow-up across multiple episodes. *Archives of General Psychiatry, 54*, 1001–1006.

Spitzer, R. L. (1983). Psychiatric diagnoses: Are clinicians still necessary? *Comprehensive Psychiatry, 24*, 399–411.

Spitzer, R. L., Williams, J. B. W., Gibbon, M., & First, M. B. (1992). The structured clinical interview for DSM-III-R (SCID): History, rationale, and description. *Archives of General Psychiatry, 49*, 624–629.

Stangl, D., Pfohl, B., Zimmerman, M., Bowers, W., & Corenthal, C. (1985). A structured interview for the DSM-III personality disorders. *Archives of General Psychiatry, 42*, 591–596.

Strober, M., Freeman, R., & Morrell, W. (1997). The long-term course of severe anorexia nervosa in adolescents: Survival analysis of recovery, relapse, and outcome predictors over 10–15 years in a prospective study. *International Journal of Eating Disorders, 22*, 339–360.

Sysko, R., Walsh, B. T., & Fairburn, C. G. (2005). EDE-Q as a measure of change in patients with bulimia nervosa. *International Journal of Eating Disorders, 37*, 100–106.

Tanofsky-Kraff, M., Morgan, C. M., Yanovski, S. Z., Marmarosh, C., Wilfley, D. E., & Yanovski, J. A. (2003). Comparison of assessment of children's eating-disordered behaviors by interview and questionnaire. *International Journal of Eating Disorders, 33*, 213–224.

Tyrer, P., Strauss, J., & Cicchetti, D. (1983). Temporal reliability of personality in psychiatric patients. *Psychological Medicine, 13*, 393–398.

Vandereycken, W., & Vanderlinden, J. (1983). Denial of illness and the use of self-reporting measures in anorexia nervosa patients. *International Journal of Eating Disorders, 2*, 101–107.

Vitousek, K. B., Daly, J., & Heiser, C. (1991). Reconstructing the internal world of the eating-disordered individual: Overcoming denial and distortion in self-report. *International Journal of Eating Disorders, 10*, 647–666.

Warshaw, M. G., Dyck, I., Allsworth, J., Stout, R. L., & Keller, M. B. (2001). Maintaining reliability in a long-term psychiatric study: An ongoing inter-rater reliability monitoring program using the longitudinal interval follow-up evaluation. *Journal of Psychiatric Research, 35*, 297–305.

Warshaw, M. G., Keller, M. B., & Stout, R. L. (1994). Reliability and validity of the Longitudinal Interval Follow-Up Evaluation for assessing outcome of anxiety disorders. *Journal of Psychiatric Research, 28*, 531–545.

Wilfley, D. E., Schwartz, M. B., Spurrell, E. B., & Fairburn, C. G. (2000). Using the eating disorder examination to identify the specific psychopathology of binge eating disorder. *International Journal of Eating Disorders, 27*, 259–269.

Williamson, D. A. (1990). *Assessment of eating disorders: Obesity, anorexia, and bulimia nervosa.* New York: Pergamon Press.

Williamson, D. A., Gleaves, D. H., & Stewart, T. M. (2005). Categorical versus dimensional models of eating disorders: An examination of the evidence. *International Journal of Eating Disorders, 37*, 1–10.

Williamson, D. A., Womble, L. G., Smeets, M. A. M., Netemeyer, R. G., Thaw, J. M., Kutlesic, V., et al. (2002). Latent structure of eating disorder symptoms: A factor analytic and taxometric investigation. American Journal of Psychiatry, 159, 412–418.

Wilson, G. T. (1993). Assessment of binge eating. In C. G. Fairburn & G. T. Wilson (Eds.), *Binge eating: Nature, assessment, and treatment* (pp. 227–249). New York: Guilford Press.

Wilson, G. T., & Smith, D. (1989). Assessment of bulimia nervosa: An evaluation of the Eating Disorder Examination. *International Journal of Eating Disorders*, *8*, 173–179.

Zanarini, M. C., Frankenburg, F. R., Chauncey, D. L., & Gunderson, J. G. (1987). The Diagnostic Interview for Personality Disorders: Interrater and test–retest reliability. *Comprehensive Psychiatry*, *28*, 467–480.

Zanarini, M. C., Frankenburg, F. R., Sickel, A. E., & Yong, L. (1996). *The Diagnostic Interview for DSM-IV Personality Disorders (DIPD-IV)*. Belmont, MA: McLean Hospital.

Zanarini, M. C., Skodol, A. E., Bender, D., Dolan, R., Sanislow, C., Schaeffer, E., et al. (2000). The Collaborative Longitudinal Personality Disorders Study: Reliability of Axis I and II diagnoses. *Journal of Personality Disorders*, *14*, 291–299.

CHAPTER 6

Self-Report Measures

Carol B. Peterson
James E. Mitchell

A large variety of self-report measures are available to assess patients with eating disorders and associated symptoms. Many have been traditionally used for research, but clinicians are increasingly finding such instruments useful in evaluating and treating patients in practice. In this chapter, we first discuss issues regarding the use of self-report measures, including their purpose, administration, and interpretation, as well as limitations related to cost, reliability, and time. We then describe some of the available measures that have been developed specifically to assess patients with eating disorders. In the final section, we review several measures of comorbid and associated features, including quality of life, mood, and personality, that may have clinical utility in working with these populations.

THE USE OF SELF-REPORT MEASURES

Several issues are important to consider regarding the use of self-report measures. Perhaps the first and most important consideration is the selection of a particular instrument for clinical or research purposes. The clinician or researcher should start by determining what data are needed and for what purpose. Self-report instruments can be used for several purposes:

- To quantify symptomatology (e.g., rating scales that measure the severity of depression).
- To verify diagnosis (e.g., measures structured to assess diagnostic criteria for certain illnesses).
- To examine specific associated clinical features (e.g., instruments that measure psychological constructs like perfectionism).
- To examine change over time. This last category can be particularly relevant in charting the success or ineffectiveness of a given intervention in research or clinical work, and can also yield useful information to provide to third-party payers.

A second important issue concerns the interpretation of instruments. Some instruments can be interpreted with simple calculations; for example, several measures of the severity of depression can be computed easily to determine an overall level of depressive symptomatology. Other measures are more complicated to score and interpret, requiring considerable time and even computer assistance. The complexity of scoring and interpretation can be costly in terms of both time and money. Financial and time burdens are particularly problematic in clinical settings because third-party payers do not usually reimburse for the use of self-report measures. Another financial consideration is the issue of copyright, because the majority of self-report measures are copyrighted and require that clinicians obtain permission and pay for their use. Although the amount for one usage is typically modest, the costs can mount over time and become a significant financial burden if patients have to pay the cost out of pocket.

The use and interpretation of self-report measures also raise potential problems for the therapeutic relationship in clinical settings. Self-report data can be extremely helpful for the clinician to determine a diagnosis and treatment plan. In addition, discussing the results of self-report data can enhance rapport and facilitate collaboration between the clinician and the patient. However, information obtained using self-report questionnaires has a number of limitations. The first type of problem involves the instrument itself. Each measure has its own strengths and weaknesses, and the clinician needs to know the validity and reliability data for specific populations that support the use of the instrument. The second type of limitation is related to the accuracy of self-report. Some patients may want to answer questions honestly but have difficulty remembering specific behavior, attitudes, or symptoms or may be influenced by cognitive biases (Schacter, 1999). Others may lack the self-awareness to answer certain types of questions, especially for complex and abstract constructs. For example, some patients are unable to consider the extent to which their self-evaluation is influenced by weight and shape. Self-report data can also be limited by patients who are trying to minimize their symptoms due to fear or anger about being forced into a treatment setting (Vitousek, Daly, & Heiser, 1991). The clinician should be aware of these limitations when using self-report data to formulate a patient's diagnosis and treatment plan. Because these instruments may communicate a greater degree of certainty than is accurate, clinicians and patients should be cautious in order to avoid overinterpreting the results.

ASSESSMENT OF SYMPTOMS OF EATING DISORDERS

The following section includes summaries of self-report questionnaires that can be used to assess eating disorder symptoms. Although a detailed review of psychometric data for each instrument is beyond the scope of this chapter, the extent to which these measures have been found to be reliable, meaning consistent internally and over time, and valid, meaning that the questionnaire accurately measures what it is intended to assess, will be summarized briefly. Questionnaires that focus more specifically on aspects of body image are described in Chapter 10.

Eating Disorder Inventory

The Eating Disorder Inventory (EDI; Garner & Olmsted, 1984; Garner, Olmsted, & Polivy, 1983) was developed as a measure of eating disorder symptoms as well as psychological variables thought to be associated with these syndromes. When it was revised, the 91-item EDI-2 retained the eight subscales from the original version (Drive for Thinness, Bulimia, Body Dissatisfaction, Ineffectiveness, Perfectionism, Interpersonal Distrust, Interoceptive Awareness, and Maturity Fears) and added three additional subscales: Asceticism, Impulse Regulation, and Social Insecurity (Garner, 1991). The EDI-2 also has a separate questionnaire that can be used as a symptom checklist (EDI-SC).

Considerable research has been conducted to support the psychometric properties of the EDI and the EDI-2. Internal consistency scores for the original eight subscales have generally been found to be greater than .80 (Garner, 1991; Garner & Olmsted, 1984; Raciti & Norcross, 1987; Wear & Pratz, 1987), and good test–retest reliability has been demonstrated (Wear & Pratz, 1987). Scores on the EDI and EDI-2 have also been observed to be relatively stable over time in longitudinal studies (Crowther, Lilly, Crawford, & Shepherd, 1992; Garner, 1991; Tasca, Illing, Lybanon-Daigle, Bissada, & Balfour, 2003). The reliability of the newer, provisional subscales is less clear (Eberenz & Gleaves, 1994; Garner, 1991). A number of studies support the validity of the EDI-2 (Garner, 1991; Gross, Rosen, Leitenberg, & Willmuth, 1986; Rathner & Rumpold, 1994; Schoemaker, van Strien, & van der Staak, 1994; Welch & Hall, 1989; Welch, Hall, & Norring, 1990), although the validity of the three provisional subscales has not been established (Eberenz & Gleaves, 1994). Several studies have found that the psychometric properties of the EDI-2 may not generalize well to other types of populations including older patients (Rofey, Shuman, Corcoran, & Birbaum, 2002), younger patients (Shore & Porter, 1990), males, (Rathner & Rumpold, 1994), and ethnically diverse samples (Franko et al., 2002; Striegel-Moore et al., 2002).

The EDI-2 can be easily administered and scored. The scoring materials include a graph with eating disorder and non-eating disorder norms that can be used for plotting results, providing a helpful illustration to patients and clinicians. The EDI-2 is a widely used measure in research settings and clinical practice and has been translated into a number of languages.

Recently, a third revision of the EDI was published (EDI-3; Garner, 2004). Although the original items have been retained, the new 91-item version includes the original three eating disorder subscales (Drive for Thinness, Bulimia, Body Dissatisfaction) as well as nine other subscales (Low Self-Esteem, Personal Alienation, Interpersonal Insecurity, Interpersonal Alienation, Interoceptive Deficits, Emotional Dysregulation, Perfectionism, Asceticism, and Maturity Fears). The scoring has been changed to include six composite scores: (1) Eating Disorder Risk, (2) Ineffectiveness, (3) Interpersonal Problems, (4) Affective Problems, (5) Overcontrol, and (6) General Psychological Maladjustment, as well as Infrequency and Negative Impression scores. Initial reliability and validity data appear to be strong (Garner, 2004), although further psychometric evaluation of the EDI-3 is necessary.

Eating Disorder Examination–Questionnaire

The Eating Disorder Examination–Questionnaire (EDE-Q; Fairburn & Beglin, 1994) was adapted from the interview version of the Eating Disorder Examination (EDE; Fairburn & Cooper, 1993), a widely used measure of eating disorder symptoms that has been described as the most accurate method of assessing binge eating (Wilson, 1993) and has considerable reliability and validity data to support its use (Fairburn & Cooper, 1993). Although the two versions of the EDE contain identical items, a number of investigations have found that the agreement between the questionnaire and interview versions is inconsistent (Black & Wilson, 1996; Carter, Aime, & Mills, 2001; Fairburn & Beglin, 1994; Passi, Bryson, & Lock, 2002; Wilfley, Schwartz, Spurrell, & Fairburn, 1997; Wolk & Walsh, 2002), especially for more complicated constructs including binge eating. Recent studies have suggested that the reliability and validity of the EDE-Q may be enhanced by providing more detailed definitions of binge eating and other concepts at the time that the questionnaire is administered (Celio, Wilfley, Crow, Mitchell, & Walsh, 2003; Goldfein et al., 2002; Passi et al., 2002). Preliminary data indicate that the EDE-Q has acceptable levels of reliability (Luce & Crowther, 1999) but further investigations are needed to establish the psychometric properties of this instrument.

The 33-item EDE-Q focuses on eating disorder symptoms and attitudes for the past 28 days and contains four subscales: Restraint, Eating Concern, Shape Concern, and Weight Concern. The subscale and total scores are based on averages from 0 to 6, with higher scores reflecting greater pathology. In addition, the measure includes questions about the frequency of symptoms including binge eating and compensatory behaviors for the past 28 days. Although the measure has been used most often in research, it can be useful in clinical settings as well.

Multiaxial Assessment of Eating Disorder Symptoms

The Multiaxial Assessment of Eating Disorder Symptoms (MAEDS; Anderson, Williamson, Duchmann, Gleaves, & Barbin, 1999) is a 56-item questionnaire designed to assess treatment outcome. The instrument contains six subscales: Binge Eating, Purgative Behavior, Avoidance of Forbidden Foods, Restrictive Eating, Fear of Fatness, and Depression. The MAEDS has been found to have excellent reliability and several studies have supported its validity (Anderson et al., 1999; Martin, Williamson, & Thaw, 2000).

Stirling Eating Disorder Scales

The Stirling Eating Disorder Scales (SEDS; Williams et al., 1994) is an 80-item instrument devised to evaluate eating disorder behavior and cognitions as well as self-esteem, assertiveness, and self-directed hostility. A preliminary investigation found that the measure demonstrated good reliability and validity (Williams et al., 1994). A recent study found that the SEDS correlated well with the EDE in an adolescent sample (Campbell, Lawrence, Serpell, Lask, & Neiderman, 2002).

Eating Disorder Questionnaire

The Eating Disorder Questionnaire (EDQ; Mitchell, Hatsukami, Eckert, & Pyle, 1985) is a measure designed to be used as a database in clinical and research settings. The EDQ includes questions about demographics, family history, weight history, medical history, and eating disorder symptoms. It also includes a timeline self-monitoring form (Eating Behaviors III) that can be used to track symptoms over time. In addition to providing extensive descriptive information, the EDQ includes questions about age of onset of symptoms and past as well as current severity. A copy of one version of the EDQ is included in Chapter 4, with a limited release of copyright to purchasers of this book for their own clinical use.

DSM-IV Diagnostic Questionnaires

Several questionnaires have been developed to establish DSM-IV diagnoses in addition to the EDI-SC (described earlier). The Eating Disorder Diagnostic Scale (EDDS; Stice, Telch, & Rizvi, 2000) is a recently developed 22-item self-report instrument designed to diagnose anorexia nervosa, bulimia nervosa, and binge eating disorder according to DSM-IV criteria. To increase the accuracy of self-reported overeating episodes, the authors of the measure purposely did not include the word *binge*, which can be misinterpreted (Beglin & Fairburn, 1992), but instead provide behavioral definitions. Preliminary investigations indicate that this measure has excellent reliability and validity, as well as diagnostic specificity and sensitivity (Stice et al., 2000; Stice, Fisher, & Martinez, 2004).

The Questionnaire for Eating Disorder Diagnoses (Q-EDD; Mintz, O'Halloran, Mulholland, & Schneider, 1997) is a 50-item self-report instrument designed for both clinicians and researchers to make DSM-IV diagnoses of bulimia nervosa and anorexia nervosa. An initial investigation supported the reliability and validity of this questionnaire (Mintz et al., 1997).

The Questionnaire on Eating and Weight Pattern–Revised (QEWP-R; Spitzer et al., 1992) contains items that allow the researcher or clinician to assign DSM-IV diagnoses for binge eating disorder and bulimia nervosa. The 28-item measure also includes questions about weight history and body image. Investigations have supported the psychometric properties of the QEWP-R to some extent (Nangle, Johnson, Carr-Nangle, & Engler, 1994; Pike, Loeb, & Walsh, 1995), although the agreement between diagnoses determined by the questionnaire compared to interviews is modest (de Zwaan et al., 1993).

Screening Instruments

Several questionnaires have been designed as screening instruments of severity and can be used in nonclinical as well as clinical samples. The Eating Attitudes Test (EAT; Garner & Garfinkel, 1979) is a 40-item measure that was developed as a screening instrument for eating disorder symptoms and has been found to have acceptable levels of reliability and validity (Garner, Olmsted, Bohr, & Garfinkel, 1982; Raciti & Norcross, 1987). A shorter version of the EAT with 26 items has also been found to correlate with other measures of eating disorder symptoms (Winnik Berland, Thompson, & Linton, 1986). Although data support its reliability and validity (Williamson, Anderson, Jackman, & Jackson, 1995), the sensitivity and specificity of the EAT as a screening instrument have been questioned (Williams, Hand, & Tarnopolsky, 1982) and it appears to have a high false-positive rate (Johnsone-Sabine, Wood, & Patton, 1988; Meadows, Palmer, Newball, & Kenrick, 1986; Mintz et al., 1997).

Based on the original measure (Smith & Thelen, 1984), the Bulimia Test–Revised (BULIT-R; Thelen, Farmer, Wonderlich, & Smith, 1991) is a 36-item questionnaire designed as a screening tool for bulimia nervosa. Studies have supported the reliability and validity of this instrument (Thelen et al., 1991; Welch, Thompson, & Hall, 1993), including its significant correlation with DSM-IV criteria (Thelen, Mintz, & Vander Wal, 1996).

The Bulimic Investigatory Test, Edinburgh (BITE; Henderson & Freeman, 1987) was designed for use in epidemiological studies as well as a measure of treatment outcome. This 33-item instrument contains a symptom subscale and a severity subscale as well as a total score. Several studies have documented the reliability of the BITE, with modest support of its validity as well (Henderson & Freeman, 1987; Waller, 1992).

The SCOFF is a 5-item screening instrument used to detect eating disorders (Morgan, Reid, & Lacey, 1999). A recent comparison of the written and interview version of this instrument found excellent agreement between the two versions (kappa coefficients = .75–.86; Perry et al., 2002), and an additional study found that the questionnaire correlated well with a clinical interview based on the DSM-IV criteria (Luck et al., 2002). Because this scale was designed in the United Kingdom, the version designed for use in the United States has not been evaluated empirically.

Binge Eating Scale

The Binge Eating Scale (BES; Gormally, Black, Daston, & Rardin, 1982) is a 16-item questionnaire developed to assess the severity of binge eating. The measure includes questions about behavioral and cognitive aspects of binge eating and provides a total severity score. Preliminary psychometric data support its internal consistency and concurrent validity (Gormally et al., 1982), and BES severity scores have been found to correlate with independent measures of binge eating in several studies (e.g., Marcus, Wing, & Hopkins, 1988; Telch & Agras, 1994).

Three-Factor Eating Questionnaire (Eating Inventory)

The Three-Factor Eating Questionnaire (TFEQ; Stunkard & Messick, 1985) is a 51-item instrument that was originally developed to measure three constructs: Restraint, Hunger, and Disinhibition. The measure has more recently been referred to as the Eating Inventory. Several investigations have not supported the original factor structure of the TFEQ (Ganley, 1988; Hyland, Irvine, Thacker, Dann, & Dennis, 1989), including a recent study that used a shortened version of the questionnaire with a large sample of twins (Mazzeo, Aggen, Anderson, Tozzi, & Bulik, 2003). Findings from other validity investigations have also been inconsistent (Eldredge & Agras, 1994; Gorman & Allison, 1995; Karlsson, Persson, Sjostrom, & Sullivan, 2000). Although the TFEQ is widely used and has been found to have good reliability (Allison, Kalinsky, & Gorman, 1992; Laessle, Tuschl, Kotthaus, & Pirke, 1989), the psychometric data supporting the validity of this instrument have not been consistent.

Measures of Dietary Restraint

In addition to the Restraint subscales of the TFEQ and EDE-Q, several other measures of dietary restraint have been developed, including the Restraint Scale (RS; Polivy, Herman, & Warsh, 1978; Ruderman, 1983) and the restraint scale of the Dutch Eating Behavior Questionnaire (van Strien, Frijters, Bergers, & Defares, 1986), both of which contain 10 items. Several studies have supported the reliability of these measures (Laessle et al., 1989; van Strien et al., 1986). However, results from several investigations have indicated that dietary restraint scores do not correlate highly with caloric restriction (Gorman & Allison, 1995; Laessle et al., 1989; Stice, Fisher, & Lowe, 2004) and the validity of both the measures and the concept of dietary restraint has been questioned (Ruderman, 1986), especially the confound between food restriction and disinhibition of dietary control (Stice, Ozer, & Kees, 1997). Critics and proponents agree that these measures are multidimensional and measure more than one construct, although results of factor-analytic studies have been inconsistent and have varied in overweight compared to nonoverweight samples (Allison et al., 1992; Gorman & Allison, 1995; Heatherton, Herman, Polivy, King, & McGree, 1988; Laessle et al., 1989; Ogden, 1993; Ruderman, 1986; van Strien, 1999).

Eating Disorder Cognitions

A number of eating disorder measures can be used to assess eating disorder cognitions, including the EDI and the EDE-Q. In addition, several questionnaires have been developed that focus exclusively on eating disorder cognitions. The Mizes Anorectic Cognitions Scale (Mizes & Klesges, 1989) is a 33-item measure to assess cognitions in anorexia nervosa as well as bulimia nervosa with established reliability and validity (Mizes, 1991, 1992; Mizes & Klesges, 1989; Williamson et al., 1995). The questionnaire was recently revised and shortened to 24 items and three subscales: Self-Control, Approval, and Fear of Weight Gain. The revised version appears to have excellent reliability and better criterion-related validity than the original measure (Mizes et al., 2000).

Several measures have been devised to assess cognitions in bulimia nervosa. Two questionnaires, the Bulimic Thoughts Questionnaire (Phelan, 1987) and the Bulimic Automatic Thoughts Test (Franko & Zuroff, 1992) each contain 20 items. The Bulimia Cognitive Distortions Questionnaire (Schulman, Kinder, Powers, Prange, & Gleghorn, 1986) is a 25-item questionnaire that assesses cognitive distortions related to eating habits and appearance. Only preliminary data are available about the reliability and validity of these three measures of cognition.

Impact of Weight on Quality of Life

The Impact of Weight on Quality of Life (IWQOL; Kolotkin, Head, Hamilton, & Tse, 1995) is a 74-item questionnaire devised to assess how body weight affects various aspects of psychosocial functioning. Several studies have supported the psychometric properties of the original questionnaire, and a more recent investigation found excellent levels of reliability and validity for a shorter version (IWQOL-Lite; Kolotkin & Crosby, 2002; Kolotkin, Crosby, Kosloski, & Williams, 2001).

ASSESSMENT OF ASSOCIATED FEATURES AND COMORBIDITY

Quality of Life

Patients with eating disorders report significant psychosocial impairment in many aspects of their lives (Crow & Peterson, 2003). For this reason, clinicians and researchers often find it informative to use questionnaires that assess quality of life. One of the most widely used quality of life measures in psychopathology research is the Social Adjustment Scale—Self-Report (SAS-SR; Weissman & Bothwell, 1976), which was derived from an interview version of the measure. The questionnaire contains 54 items that focus on recent social adjustment in different roles. It includes six subscales: Work, Extended Family, Marital, Parental, Social and Leisure, and Family Unit. The psychometric properties of the SAS-SR have been supported by a number of studies (Weissman & Bothwell, 1976; Weissman, Prusoff, Thompson, Harding, & Myers, 1978; Weissman, Olfson, Gameroff, Feder, & Fuentes, 2001).

Another measure that has been used to assess quality of life is the Short-Form 36 (SF-36; Ware, Kosinksi, & Dewey, 2000), a 36-item health measure that focuses on functioning for the past four weeks (although an acute version assessing the past week is also available). The SF-36 includes eight subscales: General Health, Physical Functioning, Role–Physical (physical limitations), Bodily Pain, Mental Health, Role–Emotional (limitations from emotional difficulties), Vitality, and Social Functioning. Scoring is norm-based. Although the SF-36 was not designed to assess quality of life among patients with psychopathology in particular, it has been widely used in psychiatric research. The reliability and validity of the SF-36 have been well established (McHorney, Ware, Lu, & Sherbourne, 1994; McHorney, Ware, & Raczek, 1993; Pukrop et al., 2003).

Depression

Comorbid mood disorders are extremely common among patients with eating disorders (Crow, Zander, Crosby, & Mitchell, 1996; Mitchell,

Specker, & de Zwaan, 1991). Used in conjunction with a diagnostic interview, self-report measures can provide useful information including the range and severity of mood disorder symptoms. Questionnaires can also be administered along with clinician-rated assessment interviews including the Hamilton Depression Rating Scale (Hamilton, 1960, 1967) or the Montgomery–Asberg Depression Rating Scale (Montgomery & Asberg, 1979). Because changes in weight and shape are included in the diagnostic criteria for major depression (American Psychiatric Association, 1994), the clinician or researcher should be cautious in interpreting these symptoms as indications of depression among patients with eating disorders.

Beck Depression Inventory

The Beck Depression Inventory (BDI; Beck, Ward, Mendelson, Mock, & Erbaugh, 1961; Beck, Rush, Shaw, & Emery, 1979) is one of the most widely used measures in research and clinical settings. It is a 21-item questionnaire that focuses on the frequency of depressive features, including mood, self-evaluation, guilt, suicidal ideation, and physical symptoms. Extensive research has been conducted that provides evidence for the reliability and validity of the BDI (Beck, Steer, & Garbin, 1988). The BDI is easy to administer and provides a total score that can be used as an indicator of depression severity.

Inventory of Depressive Symptomatology—Self-Report

The Inventory of Depressive Symptomatology—Self-Report (IDS-SR; Rush et al., 1986) contains 30 items that focus on the frequency of occurrence of physical and psychological depressive symptoms. A number of investigations have found evidence of the reliability and validity of the IDS-SR (Biggs et al., 2000; Rush et al., 1986; Rush, Gullion, Basco, Jarrett, & Trivedi, 1996; Trivedi et al., 2004). A briefer version with 16 items has recently been constructed, called the Quick Inventory of Depressive Symptomatology; this version appears to have strong psychometric properties as well (Rush et al., 2003; Trivedi et al., 2004).

Zung Self-Rating Depression Scale

The Zung Self-Rating Depression Scale (SDS; Zung, 1965; Zung, Richards, & Short, 1965) contains descriptions of 20 symptoms of depression, including affective, physiological, psychological, and psychomotor. On the SDS, the patient notes the frequency of these symptoms for the past week using a four-point scale. Like the BDI and the IDS-SR, the SDS provides a total score that can be used as a measure of depression severity. The reliability and validity of the SDS measure have been supported by a number of investigations (Lambert, Hatch, Kingston, & Edwards, 1986; Schaefer et al., 1985; Thurber, Snow, & Honts, 2002).

Inventory to Diagnose Depression

In contrast to the BDI, IDS-SR, and SDS, the Inventory to Diagnose Depression (IDD; Zimmerman, Coryell, Corenthal, & Wilson, 1986) is a 22-item measure that can be used to determine diagnosis as well as symptom severity. The IDD items ask about the presence or absence of each symptom as well as the extent to which each symptom occurred for the past two weeks. The reliability and validity of the IDD have been observed in several studies (Goldston, O'Hara, & Schartz, 1990; Zimmerman et al., 1986; Zimmerman & Coryell, 1987).

In summary, several self-report questionnaires can be used to assess the severity of depressive symptoms. The IDD measures symptom severity as well as providing diagnostic information. Most of these self-report instruments are supported by extensive psychometric data. In general, they are easy to administer and score and useful for both clinicians and researchers.

ASSESSMENT OF PERSONALITY

Personality Diagnostic Questionnaire–4

The Personality Diagnostic Questionnaire–4 (PDQ-4; Hyler, Rieder, et al. 1989; Hyler, Lyons, et al., 1990) is an 85-item true–false questionnaire designed to assess specific DSM-IV personality disorder diagnostic criteria (American Psychiatric Association, 1994). Items have been reorganized so that they no longer follow the specific personality disorder groups. This instrument assesses the 10 personality disorders included in the DSM-IV as well as passive–aggressive (negativistic) and depressive personality disorders described in Appendix B (i.e., diagnoses requiring further study). An index of overall personality disturbances is also included. Given the problem with sensitivity, many patients will meet criteria for more than one diagnosis. Comparison with semistructured clinical interviews generally shows considerable evidence of overdiagnosis by self-report.

Millon Clinical Multi-Axial Inventory–3

The Millon Clinical Multi-Axial Inventory–3 (MCMI-3; Millon, Davis & Millon, 1997) is a 175-item true–false self-report measure that includes 24 subscales, including 14 personality patterns. The instrument differentiates between clinical personality styles and what are considered severe personality pathology (i.e., schizotypal, paranoid, and borderline). It can be used to assess personality styles both dimensionally and categorically. The scale is designed to reflect Millon's theoretical model. The instrument may also exhibit high false-positive rates.

Wisconsin Personality Disorders Inventory–4

The Wisconsin Personality Disorders Inventory–4 (WISPI-4; Benjamin, 1996; Klein, et al., 1993) includes 214 items and provides both continuous and categorical scores for the 10 DSM-IV Axis II personality disorders and for passive-aggressive personality. It reflects the interpersonal perspective of Benjamin's Structural Analysis of Social Behavior (Benjamin, 1996). A computer-administered and computer-scored version is available.

NEO Personality Inventory—Revised

The NEO Personality Inventory—Revised (NEO PI-R; Costa & McCrae, 1992; Juni, 1996) is a 240-item questionnaire that yields scale scores in six domains and on six facets within each of these domains. It also includes validity items. Scores are interpreted by examining domain and facet scores compared to normative groups. This instrument assesses the five-factor model of personality traits.

Dimensional Assessment of Personality Pathology

The Dimensional Assessment of Personality Pathology (DAPP; Livesley, Jackson, & Schroeder, 1992; Goldner, Srikameswaran, Schroeder, Livesley, & Birmingham, 1999) is a 290-item self-report measure consisting of 18 scales. These 18 scales are organized into four factors: emotional dysregulation, dissocial behavior, inhibitedness, and compulsivity. The DAPP was standardized on a clinical population, which enhances its validity for clinical research. The instrument has been shown to have satisfactory psychometric properties.

SUMMARY

A number of self-report questionnaires can be used to measure behavioral and psychological aspects of eating disorders and other related constructs. Many of these instruments are supported by extensive validity and reliability data, but psychometric information about others is more preliminary. Certain eating disorder symptoms are especially challenging to measure accurately using self-report measures, especially abstract variables such as self-evaluation and features that require clinical judgment, including binge eating episodes (Beglin & Fairburn, 1992; Wilson, 1993). The accuracy of self-reported data may be enhanced by providing specific definitions of concepts along with the questionnaire (Passi et al., 2002), including examples of what would and would not be considered objectively large binge eating episodes. In selecting a self-report questionnaire or battery of measures, the clinician or researcher should consider the psychometric strength of the instrument, the extent to which the instrument assesses the variables of interest, and the potential time burden on the patient. In addition, the limitations of self-report data should be considered when using these measures for diagnosis and treatment planning.

REFERENCES

Allison, D. B., Kalinsky, L. B., & Gorman, B. S. (1992). The comparative psychometric properties of three measures of dietary restraint. *Psychological Assessment, 4*, 391–398.

American Psychiatric Association. (1994). *Diagnostic and statistical manual of mental disorders* (4th ed.). Washington, DC: Author.

Anderson, D. A., Williamson, D. A., Duchmann, E. G., Gleaves, D. H., & Barbin, J. M. (1999). Development and validation of a multifactorial treatment outcome measure for eating disorders. *Assessment, 6*, 7–20.

Beck, A. T., Rush, A. J., Shaw, B. F., & Emery, G. (1979). *Cognitive therapy of depression*. New York: Guilford Press.

Beck, A. T., Steer, R. A., & Garbin, M. G. (1988). Psychometric properties of the Beck Depression Inventory: Twenty-five years of evaluation. *Clinical Psychology Review, 8*, 77–100.

Beck, A. T., Ward, C. H., Mendelson, M., Mock, J., & Erbaugh, J. (1961). An inventory for measuring depression. *Archives of General Psychiatry, 4*, 561–571.

Beglin, S. J., & Fairburn, C. G. (1992). What is meant by the term "binge"? *American Journal of Psychiatry, 149*, 123–124.

Benjamin, L. S. (1996). *Interpersonal diagnosis and treatment of personality disorders* (2nd ed.). New York: Guilford Press.

Biggs, M. M., Shores-Wilson, K., Rush, A. J., Carmody, T. J., Trivedi, M. H., Crismon,

M. L., et al. (2000). A comparison of alternative assessments of depressive symptom severity: A pilot study. *Psychiatry Research*, 96, 269–279.

Black, C. M. D., & Wilson, G. T. (1996). Assessment of eating disorders: Interview versus questionnaire. *International Journal of Eating Disorders*, 20, 43–50.

Campbell, M., Lawrence, B., Serpell, L., Lask, B., & Neiderman, M. (2002). Validating the Stirling Eating Disorders Scales (SEDS) in an adolescent population. *Eating Behaviors*, 3, 285–293.

Carter, J. C., Aimé, A. A., & Mills, J. S. (2001). Assessment of bulimia nervosa: A comparison of interview and self-report questionnaire methods. *International Journal of Eating Disorders*, 30, 187–192.

Celio, A. A., Wilfley, D. E., Crow, S. J., Mitchell, J. E., & Walsh, B. T. (2003, May). *A comparison of the BES, QEWP-R, and EDE-Q-I with the EDE in the assessment of binge eating disorder and its symptoms*. Paper presented at the International Conference on Eating Disorders, Denver, CO.

Costa, P. T., & McCrae, R. R. (1992). NEO PI-R Professional Manual. Odessa, FL: Psychological Assessment Resources.

Crow, S. J., & Peterson, C. B. (2003). The economic and social burden of eating disorders: A review. In M. Maj, K. A. Halmi, J. J. Lopez-Ibor, & N. Sartorius (Eds.), *Evidence and experience in psychiatry: Vol. 6: Eating disorders* (pp. 385–398). London: Wiley.

Crow, S. J., Zander, K. M., Crosby, R. D., & Mitchell, J. E. (1996). Discriminant function analysis of depressive symptoms in binge eating disorder, bulimia nervosa, and major depression. *International Journal of Eating Disorders*, 19, 399–404.

Crowther, J. H., Lilly, R. S., Crawford, P. A., & Shepherd, K. L. (1992). The stability of the Eating Disorder Inventory. *International Journal of Eating Disorders*, 12, 97–101.

de Zwaan, M., Mitchell, J. E., Specker, S. M., Pyle, R. L., Mussell, M. P., & Seim, H. C. (1993). Diagnosing binge eating disorder: Level of agreement between self-report and expert-rating. *International Journal of Eating Disorders*, 14, 289–295.

Eberenz, K. P., & Gleaves, D. H. (1994). An examination of the internal consistency and factor structure of the Eating Disorder Inventory-2 in a clinical sample. *International Journal of Eating Disorders*, 16, 371–379.

Eldredge, K. L., & Agras, W. S. (1994). Instability of restraint among clinical binge eaters: A methodological note. *International Journal of Eating Disorders*, 15, 285–297.

Fairburn, C. G., & Beglin, S. J. (1994). Assessment of eating disorders: Interview or self-report questionnaire? *International Journal of Eating Disorders*, 16, 363–370.

Fairburn, C. G., & Cooper, Z. (1993). The Eating Disorder Examination (12th ed.). In C. G. Fairburn & G. T. Wilson (Eds.), *Binge eating: Nature, assessment, and treatment* (pp. 317–360). New York: Guilford Press.

Franko, D. L., Schumann, B. C., Barton, B., Daniels, S., Schreiber, G., Crawford, P., et al. (2002, November). *Stability of the factor structure of the Eating Disorders Inventory in black and white adolescent girls*. Poster presented at the Eating Disorders Research Annual Meeting, Charleston, SC.

Franko, D. L., & Zuroff, D. C. (1992). The Bulimic Automatic Thoughts Test: Initial reliability and validity data. *Journal of Clinical Psychology*, 48, 505–509.

Ganley, R. M. (1988). Emotional eating and how it relates to dietary restraint, disinhibition, and perceived hunger. *International Journal of Eating Disorders, 7*, 635–647.

Garner, D. M. (1991). *Eating Disorder Inventory–2: Professional manual.* Odessa, FL: Psychological Assessment Resources.

Garner, D. M. (2004). *Eating Disorder Inventory–3*. Lutz, FL: Psychological Assessment Resources.

Garner, D. M., & Garfinkel, P. E. (1979). The Eating Attitudes Test: An index of the symptoms of anorexia nervosa. *Psychological Medicine*, 9, 273–279.

Garner, D. M., & Olmsted, M. P. (1984). *The Eating Disorder Inventory Manual.* Odessa, FL: Psychological Assessment Resources.

Garner, D. M., Olmsted, M. P., Bohr, Y., & Garfinkel, P. E. (1982). The Eating Attitudes Test: Psychometric features and clinical correlates. *Psychological Medicine, 12*, 871–878.

Garner, D. M., Olmsted, M. P., & Polivy, J. (1983). The Eating Disorder Inventory: A measure of cognitive-behavioral dimensions of anorexia nervosa and bulimia nervosa. In P. L. Darby, P. E. Garfinkel, D. M. Garner, & D. V. Coscina (Eds.), *Anorexia nervosa: Recent developments in research* (pp. 173–184). New York: Liss.

Goldfein, J., Devlin, M., Kamenetz, C., Wolk, S., Raizman, P., & Dobrow, I. (2002, April). *EDE-Q with and without instruction to assess binge eating in patients with binge eating disorder.* Poster presented at the International Conference on Eating Disorders, Boston, MA.

Goldner, E. M., Srikameswaran, S., Schroeder, M. L., Livesley, W. J., & Birmingham, C. L. (1999) Dimensional assessment of personality pathology in patients with eating disorders. *Psychiatry Research, 85*, 151–159.

Goldston, D. B., O'Hara, M. W., & Schartz, H. A. (1990). Reliability, validity, and preliminary normative data for the Inventory to Diagnose Depression in a college population. *Psychological Assessment, 2*, 212–215.

Gormally, J., Black, S., Daston, S., & Rardin, D. (1982). The assessment of binge eating severity among obese persons. *Addictive Behaviors, 7*, 47–55.

Gorman, B. S., & Allison, D. B. (1995). Measures of restrained eating. In D. B. Allison (Ed.), *Handbook of assessment methods for eating behaviors and weight-related problems: Measures, theory, and research* (pp. 149–184). Thousand Oaks, CA: Sage.

Gross, J., Rosen, J. C., Leitenberg, H., & Willmuth, M. E. (1986). Validity of the Eating Attitudes Test and the Eating Disorders Inventory in bulimia nervosa. *Journal of Consulting and Clinical Psychology, 54*, 875–876.

Hamilton, M. (1960). A rating scale for depression. *Journal of Neurology, Neurosurgery, and Psychiatry, 23*, 56–62.

Hamilton, M. (1967). Development of a rating scale for primary depressive illness. *British Journal of Social and Clinical Psychology, 6*, 278–296.

Heatherton, T. F., Herman, C. P., Polivy, J., King, G. A., & McGree, S. T. (1988). The (mis)measurement of restraint: An analysis of conceptual and psychometric issues. *Journal of Abnormal Psychology, 97*, 19–28.

Henderson, M., & Freeman, C. P. L. (1987). A self-rating scale for bulimia: The BITE. *British Journal of Psychiatry, 150*, 18–24.

Hyland, M. E., Irvine, S. H., Thacker, C., Dann, P. L., & Dennis, I. (1989). Psychometric analysis of the Stunkard-Messick Eating Questionnaire (SMEQ) and comparison with the Dutch Eating Behavior Questionnaire (DEBQ). *Current Psychology Research and Reviews, 8*, 228–233.

Hyler, S. E., Lyons, M., Rieder, R. O., Young, L., Williams, J. B., & Spitzer, R. L. (1990) The factor structure of self-report DSM-III axis II symptoms and their relationship to clinicians' ratings. *American Journal of Psychiatry, 147*, 751–757.

Hyler, S. E., Rieder, R. O., Williams, J. B., Spitzer, R. L., Lyons, M., & Hendler, J. (1989) A comparison of clinical and self-report diagnoses of DSM-III personality disorders in 552 patients. *Comprehensive Psychiatry, 30*, 170–178.

Johnsone-Sabine, E., Wood, K., & Patton, G. (1988). Abnormal eating attitudes in London schoolgirls—A prospective epidemiological study: Factors associated with abnormal response on screening questionnaires. *Psychological Medicine, 18*, 615–622.

Juni, S. (1996). Review of the revised NEO Personality Inventory. In J. C. Conoley & J. C. Impara (Eds.), *12th Mental Measurements Yearbook* (pp. 863–868). Lincoln: University of Nebraska Press.

Karlsson, J., Persson, L. O., Sjostrom, L., & Sullivan, M. (2000). Psychometric properties and factor structure of the Three-Factor Eating Questionnaire (TFEQ) in obese men and women. *International Journal of Obesity, 24*, 1715–1725.

Klein, M. H., Benjamin, L. S., Rosenfeld, R., Treece, C., Husted, J., & Greist, J. M. (1993). The Wisconsin Personality Disorders Inventory: Development, reliability, and validity. *Journal of Personality Disorders*, (Suppl.), 18–33.

Kolotkin, R. L., & Crosby, R. D. (2002). Psychometric evaluation of the Impact of Weight on Quality of Life-Lite questionnaire (IWQOL-Lite) in a community sample. *Quality of Life Research, 11*, 157–171.

Kolotkin, R. L., Crosby, R. D., Kosloski, K. D., & Williams, G. R. (2001). Development of a brief measure to assess quality of life in obesity. *Obesity Research*, 9, 102–111.

Kolotkin, R. L., Head, S., Hamilton, M. A., & Tse, C. T. J. (1995). Assessing impact of weight on quality of life. *Obesity Research*, 3, 49–56.

Laessle, R. G., Tuschl, R. J., Kotthaus, B. C., & Pirke, K. M. (1989). A comparison of the validity of three scales for the assessment of dietary restraint. *Journal of Abnormal Psychology*, 98, 504–507.

Lambert, M. J., Hatch, D. R., Kingston, M. D., & Edwards, B. C. (1986). Zung, Beck, and Hamilton Rating Scales as measures of treatment outcome: A meta-analytic comparison. *Journal of Consulting and Clinical Psychology, 54*, 54–59.

Livesley, W. J., Jackson, D. N., & Schroeder, M. L. (1992). Factorial structure of traits delineating personality disorders in clinical and general populations. *Journal of Abnormal Psychology, 101*, 432–440.

Luce, K. H., & Crowther, J. H. (1999). The reliability of the Eating Disorder Examination—Self-report Questionnaire version (EDE-Q). *International Journal of Eating Disorders, 25*, 349–351.

Luck, A. J., Morgan, J. F., Reid, F., O'Brien, A., Brunton, J., Price, C., et al. (2002). The SCOFF questionnaire and clinical interview for eating disorders in general practice: Comparative study. *British Medical Journal, 325*, 755–756.

Marcus, M. D., Wing, R. R., & Hopkins, J. (1988). Obese binge eaters: Affect, cognitions, and response to behavioral weight control. *Journal of Consulting and Clinical Psychology*, 56, 433–439.

Martin, C. K., Williamson, D. A., & Thaw, J. M. (2000). Criterion validity of the Multiaxial Assessment of Eating Disorder Symptoms. *International Journal of Eating Disorders, 28*, 303–310.

Mazzeo, S. E., Aggen, S. H., Anderson, C., Tozzi, F., & Bulik, C. M. (2003). Investigating the structure of the Eating Inventory (Three-Factor Eating Questionnaire): A confirmatory approach. *International Journal of Eating Disorders, 34*, 255–264.

McHorney, C. A., Ware, J. E., Lu, J. F. R., & Sherbourne, C. D. (1994). The MOS 36-item Short-Form Health Survey (SF-36): III. Tests of data quality, scaling assumptions and reliability across diverse patient groups. *Medical Care, 32*, 40–66.

McHorney, C. A., Ware, J. E., & Raczek, A. E. (1993). The MOS 36-item Short-Form Health Survey (SF-36): II. Psychometric and clinical tests of validity in measuring physical and mental health constructs. *Medical Care, 31*, 247–263.

Meadows, G. N., Palmer, R. C., Newball, E. U. M., & Kenrick, J. M. T. (1986). Eating attitudes and disorders among young women: A general practice based survey. *Psychological Medicine, 16*, 351–357.

Millon, T., Davis, R., & Millon, C. (1997). *MCMI-III Manual* (2nd ed.). Minneapolis: National Computer Systems.

Mintz, L. B., O'Halloran, M. S., Mulholland, A. M., & Schneider, P. A. (1997). Questionnaire for Eating Disorder Diagnoses: Reliability and validity of operationalizing DSM-IV criteria into a self-report form. *Journal of Counseling Psychology, 44*, 63–79.

Mitchell, J. E., Hatsukami, D., Eckert, E., & Pyle, R. (1985). Eating Disorders Questionnaire. *Psychopharmacology Bulletin, 21*, 1025–1043.

Mitchell, J. E., Specker, S. M., & de Zwaan, M. (1991). Comorbidity and medical complications of bulimia nervosa. *Journal of Clinical Psychiatry, 52*(Suppl.), 13–20.

Mizes, J. S. (1991). Construct validity and factor stability of the Anorectic Cognitions Questionnaire. *Addictive Behaviors, 16*, 89–93.

Mizes, J. S. (1992). Validity of the Mizes Anorectic Cognitions Scale: A comparison between anorectics, bulimics, and psychiatric controls. *Addictive Behaviors, 17*, 283–289.

Mizes, J. S., Christiano, B., Madison, J., Post, G., Seime, R., & Varnado, P. (2000). Development of the Mizes Anorectic Cognitions Questionnaire—Revised: Psychometric properties and factor structure in a large sample of eating disorder patients. *International Journal of Eating Disorders, 28*, 415–421.

Mizes, J. S., & Klesges, R. C. (1989). Validity, reliability, and factor structure of the Anorectic Cognitions Questionnaire. *Addictive Behaviors, 14*, 589–594.

Montgomery, S. A., & Asberg, M. C. (1979). A new depression scale designed to be sensitive to change. *British Journal of Psychiatry, 134*, 382–389.

Morgan, J. F., Reid, F., & Lacey, J. H. (1999). The SCOFF questionnaire: Assessment of a new screening tool for eating disorders. *British Medical Journal, 319*, 1467–1468.

Nangle, D. W., Johnson, W. G., Carr-Nangle, R., & Engler, L. B. (1994). Binge eating disorder and the proposed DSM-IV criteria: Psychometric analysis of the Questionnaire of Eating and Weight Patterns. *International Journal of Eating Disorders, 16*, 147–157.

Ogden, J. (1993). The measurement of restraint: Confounding success and failure? *International Journal of Eating Disorders, 13*, 69–76.

Passi, V. A., Bryson, S. W., & Lock, J. (2002). Assessment of eating disorders in adolescents with anorexia nervosa: Self-report questionnaire versus interview. *International Journal of Eating Disorders, 33*, 45–54.

Perry, L., Morgan, J., Reid, F., Brunton, J., O'Brien, A., Luck, A., & Lacy, H. (2002). Screening for symptoms of eating disorders: Reliability of the SCOFF screening tool with written compared to oral delivery. *International Journal of Eating Disorders, 32*, 466–472.

Phelan, P. W. (1987). Cognitive correlates of bulimia: The Bulimic Thoughts Questionnaire. *International Journal of Eating Disorders*, 6, 593–607.

Pike, K. M., Loeb, K., & Walsh, B. T. (1995). Binge eating and purging. In D. B. Allison (Ed.), *Handbook of assessment methods for eating behaviors and weight-related problems: Measures, theory, and research* (pp. 303–346). Thousand Oaks, CA: Sage.

Polivy, J., Herman, C. P., & Warsh, S. (1978). Internal and external components of emotionality in restrained and unrestrained eaters. *Journal of Abnormal Psychology, 87*, 497–504.

Pukrop, R., Schlaak, V., Möller-Leimkühler, A. M., Albus, M., Czernik, A., Klosterkötter, J., & Möller, H. J. (2003). Reliability and validity of quality of life assessed by the Short-Form 36 and the Modular System for Quality of Life in patients with schizophrenia and patients with depression. *Psychiatry Research, 119*, 63–79.

Raciti, M. C., & Norcross, J. C. (1987). The EAT and EDI: Screening, interrelationships, and psychometrics. *International Journal of Eating Disorders*, 6, 579–586.

Rathner, G., & Rumpold, G. (1994). Convergent validity of the Eating Disorder Inventory and the Anorexia Nervosa Inventory for self-rating in an Austrian nonclinical population. *International Journal of Eating Disorders, 16*, 381–393.

Rofey, D. L., Shuman, E. S., Corcoran, K. J., & Birbaum, M. C. (2002, April). *Age matters: Internal consistency on the EDI-2.* Poster presented at the 2002 International Conference on Eating Disorders, Boston, MA.

Ruderman, A. J. (1983). The Restraint Scale: A psychometric investigation. *Behaviour Research and Therapy, 21*, 258–283.

Ruderman, A. J. (1986). Dietary restraint: A theoretical and empirical review. *Psychological Bulletin*, 99, 247–262.

Rush, A. J., Giles, D. E., Schlesser, M. A., Fulton, C. L., Weissenburger, J., & Burns, C. (1986). The Inventory for Depressive Symptomatology (IDS): Preliminary findings. *Psychiatry Research, 18*, 65–87.

Rush, A. J., Guillion, C. M., Basco, M. R., Jarrett, R. B., & Trivedi, M. H. (1996). The Inventory of Depressive Symptomatology (IDS): Psychometric properties. *Psychological Medicine*, 26, 477–86.

Rush, A. J., Trivedi, M. H., Ibrahim, H. M., Carmody, T. J., Arnow, B., Klein, D. N., et al. (2003). The 16-item Quick Inventory of Depressive Symptomatology (QIDS), Clinician Rating (QIDS-C) and Self-Report (QIDS-SR): A psychometric evaluation in patients with chronic major depression. *Biological Psychiatry, 54*, 573–583.

Schacter, D. L. (1999). The seven sins of memory: Insights from psychology and cognitive neuroscience. *American Psychologist, 54*, 182–203.

Schaefer, A., Brown, J., Watson, C. G., Plemel, D., DeMotts, J., Howard, M. T., et al. (1985). Comparison of the validities of the Beck, Zung, and MMPI depression scales. *Journal of Consulting and Clinical Psychology, 53*, 415–418.

Schoemaker, C., van Strien, T., & van der Staak, C. (1994). Validation of the Eating Disorders Inventory in a nonclinical population using transformed and untransformed responses. *International Journal of Eating Disorders, 15*, 387–393.

Schulman, R. G., Kinder, B. N., Powers, P. S., Prange, M., & Gleghorn, A. A. (1986). The development of a scale to measure cognitive distortions in bulimia. *Journal of Personality Assessment, 50*, 630–639.

Shore, R. A., & Porter, J. E. (1990). Normative and reliability data for 11 to 18 year olds on the Eating Disorder Inventory. *International Journal of Eating Disorders, 9*, 201–207.

Smith, M. C., & Thelen, M. H. (1984). Development and validation of a test for bulimia. *Journal of Consulting and Clinical Psychology, 52*, 863–872.

Spitzer, R. L., Devlin, M., Walsh, B. T., Hasin, D., Wing, R., Marcus, M., et al. (1992). Binge eating disorder: A multi-site field trial of the diagnostic criteria. *International Journal of Eating Disorders, 11*, 191–203.

Stice, E., Fisher, M., & Lowe, M. R. (2004). Are dietary restraint scales valid measures of acute dietary restriction? Unobtrusive observational data suggest not. *Psychological Assessment, 16*, 51–59.

Stice, E., Fisher, M., & Martinez, E. (2004). Eating Disorder Diagnostic Scale: Additional evidence of reliability and validity. *Psychological Assessment, 16*, 60–71.

Stice, E., Ozer, S., & Kees, M. (1997). Relation of dietary restraint to bulimic symptomatology: The effects of the criterion confounding of the Restraint Scale. *Behaviour Research and Therapy, 35*, 145–152.

Stice, E., Telch, C. F., & Rizvi, S. L. (2000). Development and validation of the Eating Disorder Diagnostic Scale: A brief self-report measure of anorexia, bulimia, and binge-eating disorder. *Psychological Assessment, 12*, 123–131.

Striegel-Moore, R. H., Franko, D. L., Barton, B. A., Schumann, B. C., Daniels, S. R., Schreiber, G. B., & Crawford, P. (2002, April). *Factor structure of the Eating Disorders Inventory*. Poster presented at the International Conference on Eating Disorders, Boston, MA.

Stunkard, A. J., & Messick, S. (1985). The Three-Factor Eating Questionnaire to measure dietary restraint and hunger. *Journal of Psychosomatic Research, 29*, 71–83.

Tasca, G. A., Illing, V., Lybanon-Daigle, V., Bissada, H., & Balfour, L. (2003). Psychometric properties of the Eating Disorders Inventory-2 among women seeking treatment for binge eating disorder. *Assessment, 10*, 228–236.

Telch, C. F., & Agras, W. S. (1994). Obesity, binge eating and psychopathology: Are they related? *International Journal of Eating Disorders, 15*, 53–61.

Thelen, M. H., Farmer, J., Wonderlich, S., & Smith, M. (1991). A revision of the Bulimia Test: The BULIT-R. *Psychological Assessment, 3*, 119–124.

Thelen, M. H., Mintz, L. B., & Vander Wal, J. S. (1996). The Bulimia Test—Revised: Validation with DSM-IV criteria for bulimia nervosa. *Psychological Assessment, 8*, 219–221.

Thurber, S., Snow, M., & Honts, C. R. (2002). The Zung Self-Rating Depression Scale: Convergent validity and diagnostic discrimination. *Assessment*, 9, 401–405.

Trivedi, M. H., Rush, A. J., Ibrahim, H. M., Carmody, T. J., Biggs, M. M., Suppes, T., et al. (2004). The Inventory of Depressive Symptomatology, Clinician Rating (IDS-C) and Self-Report (IDS-SR), and the Quick Inventory of Depressive Symptomatology, Clinician Rating (QIDS-C) and Self-Report (QIDS-SR) in public sector patients with mood disorders: A psychometric evaluation. *Psychological Medicine*, 34, 73–82.

van Strien, T. (1999). Success and failure in the measurement of restraint: Notes and data. *International Journal of Eating Disorders*, 25, 441–449.

van Strien, T., Frijters, J. E. R., Bergers, G. P. A., & Defares, P. B. (1986). The Dutch Eating Behavior Questionnaire (DEBQ) for assessment of restrained, emotional and external eating behavior. *International Journal of Eating Disorders*, 5, 295–315.

Vitousek, K. B., Daly, J., & Heiser, C. (1991). Reconstructing the internal world of the eating-disordered individual: Overcoming denial and distortion in self-report. *International Journal of Eating Disorders*, 10, 647–666.

Waller, G. (1992). Bulimic attitudes in different eating disorders: Clinical utility of the BITE. *International Journal of Eating Disorders*, 11, 73–78.

Ware, J. E., Kosinksi, M., & Dewey, J. E. (2000). *How to score Version Two of the SF-36 Health Survey*. Lincoln, RI: QualityMetric.

Wear, R. W., & Pratz, W. (1987). Test-restest reliability for the Eating Disorder Inventory. *International Journal of Eating Disorders*, 6, 767–769.

Weissman, M. M., & Bothwell, S. (1976). Assessment of social adjustment by patient self-report. *Archives of General Psychiatry*, 33, 1111–1115.

Weissman, M. M., Olfson, M., Gameroff, M. J., Feder, A., & Fuentes, M. (2001). A comparison of three scales for assessing social functioning in primary care. *American Journal of Psychiatry*, 158, 460–466.

Weissman, M. M., Prusoff, B. A., Thompson, W. D., Harding, P. S., & Myers, J. K. (1978). Social adjustment by self-report in a community sample and in psychiatric outpatients. *Journal of Nervous and Mental Disease*, 166, 317–326.

Welch, G., & Hall, A. (1989). The reliability and discriminant validity of three potential measures of bulimic behaviors. *Journal of Psychiatric Research*, 23, 125–133.

Welch, G., Hall, A., & Norring, C. (1990). The factor structure of the Eating Disorder Inventory in a patient setting. *International Journal of Eating Disorders*, 9, 79–85.

Welch, G., Thompson, L., & Hall, A. (1993). The BULIT-R: Its reliability and clinical validity as a screening tool for DSM-III-R bulimia nervosa in a female tertiary education population. *International Journal of Eating Disorders*, 14, 95–105.

Wilfley, D. E., Schwartz, M. B., Spurrell, E. B., & Fairburn, C. G. (1997). Assessing the specific psychopathology of binge eating disorder patients: Interview or self-report? *Behaviour Research and Therapy*, 35, 1151–1159.

Williams, G. J., Power, K. G., Miller, H. R., Freeman, C. P., Yellowlees, A., Dowds, T., et al. (1994). Development and validation of the Stirling Eating Disorders Scales. *International Journal of Eating Disorders*, 16, 35–43.

Williams, P., Hand, D., & Tarnopolsky, A. (1982). The problem of screening for uncommon disorders: A comment on the Eating Attitudes Test. *Psychological Medicine, 12*, 431–434.

Williamson, D. A., Anderson, D. A., Jackman, L. P., & Jackson, S. R. (1995). Assessment of eating disordered thoughts, feelings, and behaviors. In D. B. Allison (Ed.), *Handbook of assessment methods for eating behaviors and weight-related problems: Measures, theory, and research* (pp. 347–386). Thousand Oaks, CA: Sage.

Wilson, G. T. (1993). Assessment of binge eating. In C. G. Fairburn & G. T. Wilson, (Eds.), *Binge eating: Nature, assessment, and treatment* (pp. 227–249). New York: Guilford Press.

Winnik Berland, N., Thompson, J. K., & Linton, P. H. (1986). Correlation between the EAT-26 and the EAT-40, the Eating Disorders Inventory, and the Restrained Eating Inventory. *International Journal of Eating Disorders, 5*, 569–574.

Wolk, S. L., & Walsh, B. T. (2002, April). *Assessment of eating disorders in patients with anorexia nervosa: Interview versus self-report questionnaire.* Poster presented at the International Conference on Eating Disorders, Boston, MA.

Zimmerman, M., & Coryell, W. (1987). The Inventory to Diagnose Depression (IDD): A self-report scale to diagnose major depression. *Journal of Consulting and Clinical Psychology, 55*, 55–59.

Zimmerman, M., Coryell, W., Corenthal, C., & Wilson, S. (1986). A self-report scale to diagnose major depressive disorder. *Archives of General Psychiatry, 43*, 1076–1081.

Zung, W. W. K. (1965). A self-rating depression scale. *Archives of General Psychiatry, 12*, 63–70.

Zung, W. W. K., Richards, C. B., & Short, M. J. (1965). Self-rating depression scale in an outpatient clinic. *Archives of General Psychiatry, 13*, 508–515.

CHAPTER 7

Medical Assessment

Scott Crow
Susan Swigart

Careful medical assessment is a critical aspect of the clinical approach to a patient with an eating disorder. Ongoing medical assessments are also important in the care of many patients as treatment proceeds. By the time a patient presents for treatment, usually there has been a prolonged period of binge eating and purging behavior, marked weight loss, or both. These behaviors carry substantial risk for medical complications, necessitating a careful workup. Furthermore, risks associated with treatment (e.g., refeeding hypophosphatemia) require careful attention both at the beginning of and intermittently during therapy. Documentation of medical problems is important not only to allow for their effective monitoring and treatment, but in some settings (e.g., currently in the United States) the documentation of such medical complications may be critical to obtaining insurance permission for treatment sufficiently intense to meet the patient's needs.

As patients progress through treatment to remission and recovery, the burden of medical compliances typically diminishes. Whether ongoing, intermittent medical assessments are indicated for patients in recovery (e.g., for osteoporosis) remains unclear.

In this chapter we review and recommend approaches to the medical assessment of patients presenting for treatment, and for those patients who are in the midst of treatment. We discuss three broad clinical situations: low-weight patients, patients with purging behavior with or without binge eating, and obese patients with binge eating but no purging. (Clearly, though, some of these behaviors may occur in the same patient.) Finally, we discuss the potential need for ongoing medical monitoring in remitted and recovered patients.

LOW-WEIGHT PATIENTS

In many respects, the patient presenting at low weight is in the most critical need of medical assessment of any individual with an eating disorder. The requirement to assess this group carefully is underscored by these patients' extraordinarily high mortality rate (Harris & Barraclough, 1998). This assessment can accomplish several things. First, a thorough medical assessment at the onset of treatment can identify medical complications requiring specific attention (in addition to the general intervention of treating the eating disorder). For some individuals these complications can be fatal, so medical assessment can at times be lifesaving. Further, most patients at low weight present with substantial ambivalence about treatment; the presence of medical complications is often a major factor supporting their decision to enter treatment. This is true not only for the identified patient but also for family members and in some systems for third-party payers.

A standard initial assessment for patients entering treatment at low weight should include the following:

- Complete blood count
- Electrolyte battery (including phosphorus, calcium, and magnesium)
- Electrocardiogram
- Liver function tests
- Dual-energy X-ray absorptiometry (DEXA)

These assessments are selected to detect many of the more common medical complications, and in particular to try to identify those individuals at risk for serious medical compromise or even death. Blood pressure and pulse should be documented in patients who restrict intake, as well as those with purging behaviors. Dehydration in these patients may lead to orthostatic hypotension. Both for patients with restrictive behavior and for those with purging, electrolyte disturbance is a common phenomenon that must be assessed. It has been clearly demonstrated that a wide variety of electrolyte abnormalities are seen both in bulimia nervosa (BN) and anorexia nervosa (AN) (Greenfield, Mickley, Quinlan, & Roloff, 1995); these may include hypochloremia, hypokalemia, and hyponatremia. Of particular concern is hypophosphatemia (Ornstein, Golden, Jacobson, & Shenker, 2003). Patients with restrictive eating often have normal or near normal serum phosphorus at the time they present for treatment but are actually total body phosphorus depleted (this is to some extent masked by the nature of metabolic changes that occur during extreme starvation). As treatment begins, provision of adequate calories can be associated with a marked drop in serum phosphorus, sometimes to dangerous levels, requiring oral and at times intravenous repletion. This refeeding hypophosphatemia has been associated with mortality (Kohn, Golden, & Shenker, 1998); it has primarily been reported in hospital settings (Ornstein et al., 2003) but also in outpatients (Winston & Wells, 2002). Documenting initial phosphorus levels is critical and all patients should continue to be monitored during refeeding.

Several other laboratory studies are typically obtained to detect or prevent complications. A variety of hematological effects, including anemia, thrombocytopenia, and leukopenia, may be seen and can be assessed through a complete blood count. Patients with extreme self-starvation also often present with elevated liver function tests (Mickley, Greenfeld, Quinlan, Roloff, & Zwas, 1996) and these, too, should be measured.

In many settings, the degree of derangement of cardiac function plays a prominent role in decisions about level of care. In addition, it appears that a substantial number of those who die from AN suffer a catastrophic, presumably dysrhythmic cardiac event (Isager, Brinch, Kreiner, & Tolstrup, 1985). Less frequently, patients with eating disorders patients will present with chest pain symptoms (Birmingham et al., 2003) although this may be more common in patients with binge eating and purging than in those with purely restrictive behavior. Abnormalities of cardiac conduction can be observed (Cooke et al., 1994; Swenne & Larsson, 1999). For all these reasons, an electrocardiogram is a useful tool in the initial assessment.

It is widely recognized that a lengthy period of semistarvation or starvation depresses resting metabolic rate (Salisbury, Levine, Crow, & Mitchell, 1995); this can be estimated using indirect calorimetry, although such measurements are rarely of great clinical utility and are frequently omitted from the initial assessment.

Finally, another aspect of the initial assessment for selected patients includes documentation of osteopenia and/or osteoporosis through the use of dual-energy X-ray absorptiometry (DEXA). DEXA is frequently recommended for individuals who have had at least 24 months of amenorrhea in association with restrictive eating patterns (Treasure & Serpell, 2001); thus, it is a frequent part of the assessment for patients who continue in treatment, as described later in this chapter, but these same criteria may apply to a certain number of individuals even at the time they present for treatment.

PATIENTS WITH BINGE EATING AND PURGING BEHAVIORS

Assessments for patients with purging should include the following:

- Electrolyte battery
- Dental evaluation

The most commonly recognized complication to be assessed in patients with purging behavior is that of electrolyte disturbance. Earlier work has suggested that a variety of types of electrolyte disturbance are particularly common among patients with purging behavior (Greenfield et al., 1995; Crow, Salisbury, Crosby, & Mitchell, 1997). Perhaps most worrisome of these is potassium depletion. Hypokalemia has been shown to be a relatively insensitive but highly specific marker for vomiting behavior (Crow et al., 1997). In patients who abuse laxatives, low levels of magnesium and phosphorus may be more common. A full electrolyte battery is a standard part of the assessment of all purging patients.

Patients induce purging using a variety of methods, including manual stimulation of the gag reflex using a finger, a toothbrush, or other implement; many patients at more advanced stages in the illness develop the ability to vomit reflexively. A small number of patients use syrup of ipecac to induce vomiting, and the active ingredient in ipecac, emetine, can be myotoxic to both skeletal and cardiac muscle (Palmer & Guay, 1986). If careful history taking reveals the use of frequent doses of ipecac, assessment of cardiac function is indicated.

One common oral complication of vomiting behavior is parotid hypertrophy. Such bilateral painless swelling of the parotid glands is encountered fairly frequently and often appears in a relatively consistent, stereotypical fashion from patient to patient. Parotid hypertrophy may persist for months following cessation of purging (Ogren, Huerter, Pearson, Antonson, & Moore, 1987). In cases where other pathology is suspected, it may be useful to test amylase levels (using a fractionated test to differentiate pancreatic from salivary sources). Further assessment of parotid hypertrophy is typically not indicated (Kaplan, 1987).

The second common type of oral complications are dental. These can include dental caries and dental enamel erosion, particularly on the lingual surfaces of the teeth (Little, 2002). In instances where frequent vomiting behavior is reported, dental evaluation may be useful in looking for caries and documenting the extent of dental damage.

Finally, a limited number of patients with purging behavior complain of symptoms of gastrointestinal bleeding, including such symptoms as the vomiting of blood to coffee ground emesis, the passing of melanotic stools, or blood in stools. A variety of pathologies can occur, including esophageal tears, gastric erosions, hemorrhoids, and in very rare instances gastric rupture (Cuellar & Van Thiel, 1986). The extent of workup indicated is typically driven by the nature of the patient's bleeding symptoms and the potential pathologies associated with such presenting symptoms. For example, for the patient vomiting substantial amounts of blood, urgent or emergency evaluation may be indicated, whereas for patients with limited amounts of blood in stool, conservative management with assessment for anemia but without invasive evaluation may be more appropriate.

RECURRING ASSESSMENTS IN SYMPTOMATIC PATIENTS

What about the continued assessment of patients who are in treatment but have continuing symptoms (low weight, binge eating, or purging)? The answer to this question is not clear and has received little attention. The risk for hypophosphatemia in the early phase of inpatient refeeding for AN (and also perhaps outpatient refeeding) has already been described. However, as refeeding progresses, at least in the first days or perhaps weeks, the risk for hypophosphatemia may increase, even in outpatients (Ornstein et al., 2003; Winston & Wells, 2003). A switch in available energy substrates occurs with the provision of adequate nutrition, which increases the demand for phosphorus and may unmask previously undetected total-body phosphorus depletion. For this reason, repeated measurements of phosphorus are necessary early in treatment.

A second question concerns the frequency with which electrolytes should be measured in patients that continue to have purging behavior. This too is somewhat unclear. Previous work suggests that hypokalemia is not strongly associated with purging severity (Crow et al., 1997). In other words, the frequency with which someone reports purging behavior may not help predict their likelihood of having hypokalemia. In light of this, periodic electrolyte determinations in symptomatic patients is probably reasonable, particularly in those who have shown a proneness to hypokalemia in the past. Existing data do not allow firm recommendations about the frequency with which this should be measured. Similarly, existing treatment guidelines such as those of the National Institute for Clinical Excellence (2004) or the American Psychiatric Association (2000) do not include such recommendations.

The third issue to consider in patients in treatment is that of the assessment (or repeated assessment) of bone mineral density using DEXA. Such assessment is frequently recommended for patients with a 24-month or more history of amenorrhea along with restrictive eating behavior. Since bone mineral loss in AN can be progressive (Bachrach, Guido, Katzman, Litt, & Marcus, 1990; Goebel, Schweiger, Kruger, & Fichter, 1999; Herzog et al., 1993), and is associated with increased fracture risk (Lucas, Melton, Crowson, & O'Fallon, 1999), repeated assessment using DEXA appears to be indicated. Again, existing data do not allow for firm recommendations regarding frequency.

OBESE PATIENTS WITH BINGE EATING

Among community samples, binge eating disorder as defined by the currently used diagnostic entity, is among the most common of eating disorder presentations. In obese individuals, it often occurs in combination with other conditions. Some evidence suggests that the presence of binge eating in obese individuals with type 2 diabetes mellitus may be associated with a worse course of diabetes (Mannucci et al., 2002; Goodwin, Hoven, & Spitzer, 2003); apart from that, little evidence presently suggests that binge eating in this group has its own unique complications (Bulik, Sullivan, & Kendler, 2002). Rather, the medical issues requiring assessment in this group appear to be those associated with overweight and obesity; guidelines exist for such assessments (e.g., see National Task Force on the Prevention and Treatment of Obesity, 2002).

ASSESSMENT OF RECOVERED PATIENTS

Essentially no attention has been paid to the question of whether specific medical issues should be monitored in individuals with a history of eating disorder who are in long-term recovery. Of the identified potential medical complications of eating disorders, it seems likely that the great majority resolve with prolonged cessation of disordered eating and the restoration of adequate nutrition and body weight. One exception to this may be osteoporosis. Because it is so common among individuals with AN, it seems reasonable to continue to intermittently monitor for osteoporosis with DEXA. At present, effective treatments for AN-related osteoporosis have yet to be identified (Mehler, 2003). Once these are available, the urgency of osteoporosis case-finding in recovered patients will increase.

SUMMARY

A targeted medical assessment is indicated for anyone beginning treatment for eating disorders; the nature of the assessment is dictated by the presence or absence of low weight or dietary restriction, purging behaviors, and obesity, and to some extent by the duration and frequency of symptoms. Patients who continue to be symptomatic will require continued assessment; whether long-recovered patients need any specific assessment is unclear.

REFERENCES

American Psychiatric Association. (2000). Practice guideline for the treatment of patients with eating disorders. *American Journal of Psychiatry, 157*(1, Suppl.).

Bachrach, L. K., Guido, D., Katzman, D., Litt, I. F., & Marcus, R. (1990). Decreased bone density in adolescent girls with anorexia nervosa. Pediatrics, 86, 440–447.

Birmingham, C. L., Lear, S. A., Kenyon, J., Chan, S. Y., Mancini, G. B., & Frohlich, J. (2003). Coronary atherosclerosis in anorexia nervosa. *International Journal of Eating Disorders, 34*(3), 375–377.

Bulik, C. M., Sullivan, P. F., & Kendler, K. S. (2002). Medical and psychiatric morbidity in obese women with and without binge eating. *International Journal of Eating Disorders, 32,* 72–78.

Cooke, R. A., Chambers, J. B., Singh, R., Todd, G. J., Smeeton, N. C., Treasure, J., et al. (1994). QT interval in anorexia nervosa. *British Heart Journal, 72,* 69–73.

Crow, S. J., Salisbury, J. J., Crosby, R. D., & Mitchell, J. E. (1997). Serum electrolytes as markers of vomiting in bulimia nervosa. *International Journal of Eating Disorders, 21*(1), 95–98.

Cuellar, R. E., & Van Thiel, D. H. (1986). Gastrointestinal complications of the eating disorders anorexia nervosa and bulimia nervosa. *American Journal of Gastroenterology, 81,* 1113–1124.

Goebel, G., Schweiger, U., Kruger, R., & Fichter, M. M. (1999). Predictors of bone mineral density in patients with eating disorders. *International Journal of Eating Disorders, 25*, 143–150.

Goodwin, R. D., Hoven, C. W., & Spitzer, R. L. (2003). Diabetes and eating disorders in primary care. *International Journal of Eating Disorders, 33*, 85–91.

Greenfeld, D., Mickley, D., Quinlan, D. M., & Roloff, P. (1995). Hypokalemia in outpatients with eating disorders. *American Journal of Psychiatry, 152*, 60.

Harris, E. C., & Barraclough, B. (1998). Excess mortality of mental disorder. *British Journal of Psychiatry, 173*, 11–53.

Herzog, W., Minne, H., Deter, C., Leidig, G., Schelberg, D., Waster, C., et al. (1993). Outcome of bone mineral density in anorexia nervosa patients 11.7 years after first admission. *Journal of Bone Mineral Research, 8*, 597–605.

Isager, T., Brinch, M., Kreiner, S., & Tolstrup, K. (1985). Death and relapse in anorexia nervosa: Survival analysis of 151 cases. *Journal of Psychiatric Research, 19*, 515–521.

Kaplan, A. S. (1987). Hyperamylasemia and bulimia: A clinical review. *International Journal of Eating Disorders, 6*, 537–543.

Kohn, M. R., Golden, N. H., & Shenker, I. R. (1998) Cardiac arrest and delirium: Presentations of the refeeding syndrome in severely malnourished adolescents with anorexia nervosa. *Journal of Adolescent Health, 22*, 239.

Little, J. W. (2002). Eating disorders: Dental implications. *Oral Surgery Oral Medicine Oral Pathology, 93*, 138–143.

Lucas, A. R., Melton, L. J., Crowson, C. S., & O'Fallon, W. M. (1999). Long-term fracture risk among women with anorexia nervosa. *Mayo Clinic Proceedings, 74*, 972–977.

Mannucci, E., Tesi, F., Ricca, V., Pierazzuloi, E., Barciulli, E., Moretti, S., et al. (2002). Eating behavior in obese patients with and without type 2 diabetes mellitus. *International Journal of Obesity, 26*, 848–853.

Mehler, P. S. (2003). Osteoporosis in anorexia nervosa: Prevention and treatment. *International Journal of Eating Disorders, 33*, 113–126.

Mickley, D., Greenfeld, D., Quinlan, D. M., Roloff, P., & Zwas, F. (1996). Abnormal liver enzymes in outpatients with eating disorders. *International Journal of Eating Disorders, 20*, 325–329.

National Institute for Clinical Excellence. (2004). *Eating disorders: Core interventions in the treatment and management of anorexia nervosa, bulimia nervosa and related eating disorders*. London: National Institute for Clinical Excellence.

National Task Force on the Prevention and Treatment of Obesity. (2002). Medical care for obese patients: Advice for health care professionals. *American Family Physician, 65*(1), 81–88.

Ogren, F. P., Huerter, J. V., Pearson, P. H., Antonson, C. W., & Moore, C. F. (1987). Transient salivary gland hypertrophy in bulimics. *Laryngoscope, 97*, 951–953.

Ornstein, R. M., Golden, N. H., Jacobson, M. S., & Shenker, I. R. (2003). Hypophosphatemia during nutritional rehabilitation in anorexia nervosa: Implications for refeeding and monitoring. *Journal of Adolescent Health, 32*, 83–88.

Palmer, E. P., & Guay, A. T. (1986). Reversible myopathy secondary to abuse of ipecac in patients with major eating disorders. *New England Journal of Medicine, 313*, 1457–1459.

Salisbury, J. J., Levine, A. S., Crow, S. J., & Mitchell, J. E. (1995). Refeeding, metabolic rate, and weight gain in anorexia nervosa: A review. *International Journal of Eating Disorders, 17*(4), 337–346.

Swenne, I., & Larsson, P. T. (1999). Heart risk associated with weight loss in anorexia nervosa and eating disorders: Risk factors for QTc interval prolongation and dispersion. *Acta PædiatricaActa Paedat, 88*, 304–309.

Treasure, J., & Serpell, L. (2001). Osteoporosis in young people. *Psychiatric Clinics of North America, 24*, 359–370.

Winston, A. P., & Wells, F. E. (2002). Hypophosphatemia following self-treatment for anorexia nervosa. *International Journal of Eating Disorders, 32*, 245–248.

CHAPTER 8

Nutritional Assessment

Cheryl L. Rock

Altered nutritional status in patients with eating disorders results from the abnormal eating patterns and cognitive distortions related to food and weight that are the core features of these disorders. Because eating patterns and associated behaviors vary a great deal across these disorders and individuals, nutritional status and resulting problems exhibit considerable heterogeneity. Nonetheless, a framework for conducting and interpreting the nutritional assessment of these patients can be useful. This aspect of assessment is a key component of diagnosis as it enables monitoring of the effects of intervention. In addition, it may contribute to the early identification of a developing eating disorder or an individual at risk, and thus may play a role in prevention.

Many individuals, especially young women, engage in pathological dieting behaviors without meeting the current diagnostic criteria for an eating disorder and may be regarded as having subclinical eating disorders. The clinical eating disorders are only the most extreme form of pathological eating attitudes and behaviors. As a continuum of dieting and weight concerns, a spectrum of eating pathology likely exists in the general population (Fairburn & Beglin, 1990). Notably, evidence for this continuum can be found in the nutritional status and dietary patterns of the general population of college-age women (Rock, Gorenflo, Drewnowski, & Demitrack, 1996).

Components of nutritional assessment include measures of anthropometric characteristics and body composition, biochemical indicators and biological markers, and dietary assessment. Data from these various sources are evaluated collectively to describe nutritional status, define risk for resulting comorbidities, and develop the appropriate interventions. However, a few general considerations affect the interpretation of these data in this target population.

Body mass index (BMI, calculated as weight [kg]/height [m^2]) is correlated with total body fat content and is currently the recommended clinical approach to defining degree of underweight or obesity in adults (Expert Panel on the Identification, Evaluation, and Treatment of Overweight in Adults, 1998). Table 8.1 lists the general categories and definitions. BMI should be considered an indicator rather than a specific measure of adiposity. Compared with body composition measurements, such as those obtained with dual-energy X-ray absorptiometry (DEXA), BMI has been found to correlate better with total body fat at the ends of the spectrum than in the mid-range in adults (Curtin, Morabia, Pichard, & Slosman, 1997). DEXA is an imaging technique that uses a whole body scanner and two different low-dose X-rays to measure soft tissue and bone mass. This approach is considered the best one currently available for measuring body composition because it is based on a three-component model of composition, and thus, is less affected by the assumption of chemical constancy that underlies and confounds other methods.

Similar BMI cutpoints have been suggested for identifying likelihood of overweight and obesity in children and adolescents (Dietz & Bellizzi, 1999). However, using a BMI above the 85th percentile for age and sex as an index for overweight, and a BMI above the 95th percentile as an index for excess adiposity, has been the standard approach used in children (Yanovski, 2001). Weight should be measured with the patient wearing a

TABLE 8.1. Underweight, Overweight, and Obesity as Defined by Body Mass Index

Classification	BMI (weight [kg]/height [m^2])
Underweight	< 18.5
Normal	18.5–24.9
Overweight	25.0–29.9
Obesity	30.0–39.9
Extreme obesity	≥ 40

Note. Data from Expert Panel on the Identification, Evaluation, and Treatment of Overweight in Adults (1998).

hospital gown, and height obtained with the patient standing against a wall or with a stadiometer, for the most accurate measures.

Biochemical measures of nutrients or other dietary constituents can contribute to nutritional assessment and monitoring. However, the usefulness of biochemical indicators of nutritional status is based on knowledge of the physiological and other determinants of the measure.

Circulating concentrations of secretory proteins that are often used as laboratory markers of overall nutritional status (serum albumin, prealbumin [transthyretin], transferrin, and retinol-binding protein) are influenced by several dietary, metabolic, and other factors, in addition to energy balance. For example, the state of hydration of the patient when the blood sample was collected will affect these levels, and some degree of dehydration is common in anorexia nervosa (AN) and bulimia nervosa (BN). Thus, these clinical laboratory measures may not accurately reflect nutritional status or energy balance in patients with eating disorders. The circulating level of insulin-like growth factor I (IGF-I) has been suggested to be an alternative nutritional marker in patients with eating disorders (Caregaro et al., 2001), because IGF-I is affected in part by the energy balance. However, several genetic and nongenetic factors have been shown to be associated with variations in plasma IGF-I in premenopausal women (Jernstrom et al., 2001), and the sensitivity and specificity of this proposed nutritional marker have not been established.

For several micronutrients, the concentration of the nutrient in the circulating body pool (i.e., serum, plasma) is a reasonably accurate reflection of overall status. However, the amounts of some micronutrients in the circulating pool (e.g., plasma retinol or vitamin A) are homeostatically regulated and do not reflect overall status except during conditions of extreme and prolonged dietary inadequacy, or may be unrelated to intake, and thus have little relationship with total body reserves or overall status. Knowledge of the influencing nondietary factors is particularly important for accurate interpretation of the nutrient concentration in blood samples or tissues. For example, tocopherols and carotenoids are transported in the circulation nonspecifically by the cholesterol-rich lipoproteins (Rock, 1997), so lower concentrations of these lipoproteins are predictive of lower concentrations of the associated micronutrients in the circulation, independent of dietary intake or total body pool. Smoking and alcohol consumption need to be considered in the interpretation of serum and other tissue concentrations of several micronutrients, particularly compounds that may be subject to oxidation (e.g., vitamin C, tocopherols, carotenoids, folate). Medications can influence the distribution of nutrients in various body pools, in addition to influencing metabolism. Knowledge of the relationship between the indicator and the risk of nutrient depletion, in addition to the responsiveness of the indicator to interventions or change, is also necessary (Habicht & Pelletier, 1990). For some nutrients, such as calcium and zinc, a specific sensitive biomarker of diet or biochemical status indicator simply has not yet been identified.

Table 8.2 lists several examples of biochemical measures of micronutrients that may be useful as a component of nutritional assessment or monitoring of dietary intake. An important concept is that a static measurement (i.e., serum concentration) is typically not as sensitive as a functional marker in the assessment of status. Functional measures, such as the in vitro activity of an erythrocyte-derived enzyme with and without the micronutrient cofactor, will more directly reflect the overall body function relating to the nutrient. However, a good functional measure is still lacking in many instances, or the extra effort involved in the procedure limits the ability to use the functional measure in most clinical settings.

In the clinical setting, dietary intake data are typically collected via food records, dietary recalls, or diet history. Numerous studies have consistently demonstrated that self-reported dietary intakes are rarely accurate, with energy intake typically underreported in the general population by 10–30%. Further, a number of factors differentially affect the degree of misreporting, including gender, age, BMI, psychosocial and personality characteristics (e.g., social desirability), ethnicity and racial group, and body dissatisfaction (Horner et al., 2002; Novotny et al., 2003; Taren et al., 1999). Over- or underreporting is characteristic of individuals over time or by different assessment methods (Black & Cole, 2001), although each method of assessment has characteristic sources of bias. Nutrient deficiency cannot be diagnosed on the basis of dietary inadequacy; instead, these data only contribute to the overall nutritional assessment.

Keeping food records generally promotes a change in eating patterns, which explains the usefulness of food records in behavioral interventions aimed at healthy weight management. Additionally, individuals reduce the number of foods and snacks consumed and decrease the complexity of their diets by substituting foods that are simpler to record (Rebro, Patterson, Kristal, & Cheney, 1998). An alternative approach often used in research studies is to collect multiple 24-hour dietary recalls to characterize intakes (Jonnalagadda et al., 2000). This approach involves randomly selecting several days over a defined period (e.g., 3 weeks) and obtaining detailed information about which foods were eaten and the eating patterns on those days. This approach is less likely to alter the usual intake patterns during the collection period. Three or four 24-hour dietary

TABLE 8.2. Biological Indicators Useful in Nutritional Assessment or Monitoring Intakes

Nutrient	Characteristics	Comments[a]
Vitamin E: Alpha-tocopherol, plasma or serum	Varies directly with vitamin E (alpha-tocopherol) intake; slow tissue turnover and relatively large body pool	Influenced by cholesterol-carrying lipoprotein levels, smoking status
Vitamin D: 25-hydroxyitamin D, plasma or serum	Good biochemical indicator of overall vitamin D status (intake plus endogenously synthesized in response to sun exposure)	Influenced by sun exposure in addition to dietary intake of vitamin D
Vitamin C, plasma or serum	Varies directly with vitamin C intake only up to a threshold	Influenced by smoking status
Folate, whole blood or erythrocyte	Acceptable biochemical indicator of long-term folate status	Influenced by smoking status; hemoglobin measurement necessary for interpretation of results
Vitamin B6: Pyridoxal-5-phosphate, plasma	Acceptable biochemical indicator of vitamin B6 status	Influenced by circulating albumin concentration, exercise, and protein and carbohydrate intakes
Vitamin B12, plasma or serum	Not the first biochemical change that occurs in response to dietary vitamin B12 deficiency, but a definitive indicator of prolonged vitamin B12 inadequacy	Low concentrations can result from several physiologic abnormalities (i.e., pernicious anemia, atrophic gastritis, hypochlorhydria, gastric surgery) in addition to dietary inadequacy
Ferritin, serum	Considered the most sensitive and specific indicator of overall iron status	Reference (normal) ranges vary depending on method used

Note. Good or acceptable biochemical indicators of status have been established for several nutrients not on this list, but the effort involved in the analytic procedures precludes usefulness in most clinical settings. Also not listed are several nutrients (i.e., zinc, copper, calcium) for which serum or plasma concentrations are easily measured but strongly influenced by nondietary factors, and substantial additional information is needed for accurate interpretation. Food and Nutrition Board (1997, 1998, 2000, 2001).

[a]Includes additional measures needed to be obtained concurrently for interpretation, and other factors crucial in the usefulness of values obtained.

recalls may be adequate to capture usual intakes of macronutrients (protein, carbohydrate, and fat) because these nutrients have numerous food sources that are commonly consumed, and thus, less likelihood of large day-to-day variability. Accurate reflection of overall intakes of several micronutrients is less likely with only a few days of recall because these nutrients are provided by fewer foods that may be consumed more episodically (Nelson, Black, Morris, & Cole, 1989). Day-to-day variability can be especially important when assessing intakes with diet recalls in patients who exhibit marked dichotomous eating patterns (e.g., binge vs. nonbinge meals or days).

A diet history is basically a comprehensive interview that elicits descriptions of usual meals and snacks, portion sizes, frequency of food consumption across food groups, and frequency of deviations. This approach is less standardized and is not readily linked with a nutrient content database, although quantitative data based on the subjective information about usual intake can be derived.

To increase the accuracy of dietary data collected in the clinical setting, a few general strategies are recommended. When dietary data are being elicited or reviewed with a patient, a nonjudgmental and accepting demeanor is crucial. Avoid the use of terms that carry meaning or suggest judgment or expectations, and thus, inadvertently affect the patient's response; for example, ask "What was the first thing that you ate or drank after getting up?" rather than "What did you eat for breakfast?" Having measurement aids available during the interview, such as measuring cups and spoons, may improve portion size estimation. Examples of items or objects that are equivalent to a given amount of food also can help patients estimate amounts that were consumed (e.g., a deck of cards is roughly equivalent to 3 ounces of meat or fish). Table 8.3 lists examples of objects and approximately equivalent amounts of various foods.

ANOREXIA NERVOSA

As defined by the diagnostic criteria, patients with AN present with a very low weight for height, with marked reductions in both adipose tissue stores and lean body mass. The criteria specify a body weight < 85% of that expected based on age and height (with the latter typically interpreted as being a BMI < 17.5 kg/m^2 in adults) (American Psychiatric Association, 1994). The use of a pediatric growth chart permits identification of young patients who have failed to gain weight and who have growth retardation. In contrast with the patient who is underweight due

TABLE 8.3. Objects Useful for Estimating Portions in Dietary Assessment

Foods and amounts	Objects
Ice cream or frozen yogurt, ½ cup Medium potato, one	Computer mouse
Slice of bread, one	CD case
Bagel, regular size	Hockey puck
Meat or fish, 1 ounce	Matchbox
Meat or fish, 3 ounces	Deck of playing cards Bar of soap Checkbook
Meat or fish, 8 ounces	Thin paperback book
Cheese, 1 ounce	Dice, four
Mashed potatoes, 1 cup Cooked rice, 1 cup Cooked pasta, 1 cup	Fist Tennis ball
Tofu, 3½ ounces	Ice cubes, four
Peanut butter, 2 tablespoons	Ping Pong ball

to a condition such as infection or malabsorption, low body weight in the patient with AN is the result of a purposeful effort to lose weight and maintain low weight by limiting energy intake, increasing energy expenditure, or both, typically over a period of months. This pattern of weight loss enables metabolic adaptations that affect the interpretation of biochemical and other indicators of malnutrition.

Several methods to measure body composition in these patients are available and have been examined in numerous research studies, and as noted earlier, DEXA is currently considered the best method. If this technology is not available, estimations based on skinfold measurements (when performed by trained individuals) have been shown to be an acceptable alternative (Kerruish et al., 2002; Probst, Goris, Vandereycken, & Van Coppenolle, 2001). Accumulation of extracellular water, which typically occurs during refeeding, limits the usefulness of body composition measures that rely on estimates of body water as a predictor of lean body mass (i.e., bioelectric impedance) (Krahn, Rock, Dechert, Nairn, & Hasse, 1993; Vaisman, Corey, Rossi, Goldberg, & Pencharz, 1988).

During weight restoration, both fat and lean body mass are regained, with fat accounting for approximately 48–68% of the gain in total body mass (Grinspoon et al., 2001; Krahn et al., 1993; Probst et al., 2001; Russell, Mira, et al., 1994). Although fat (particularly trunk fat) may account for a somewhat greater proportion of the weight gained during treatment, the weight-restored or recovered patient still has a lower amount of body fat than healthy control subjects (Russell et al., 1994; Wentz et al., 2003).

Clinical laboratory data that typically relate to nutritional factors in the general population must be interpreted within the context of the neuroendocrine and other physiological abnormalities present in AN (Becker, Grinspoon, Kubanski, & Herzog, 1999; Gold et al., 1986). For example, hypercholesterolemia, if present, is a consequence of thyroid abnormalities in response to severe dietary restriction. Circulating concentrations of the secretory proteins (e.g., serum albumin) are typically normal or low-normal at diagnosis, depending in part on the state of hydration and the severity of the weight loss. Although within the normal range at admission, an increase in serum prealbumin concentration has been observed in response to treatment and weight restoration in patients with AN in one case series report (Castro, Deulofeu, Gila, Puig, & Toro, 2004). Hypercarotenemia is often present in these patients due to the consumption of high-carotenoid foods (i.e., deeply pigmented vegetables and fruits) by low-weight individuals (Mazzone & Dal Canton, 2002; Rock & Swendseid, 1993), and is innocuous. Carotenoid absorption is inefficient but unregulated, so peripheral tissue concentrations are largely determined by intake versus relative body mass and tissue capacity. An individual with a smaller body mass has a higher tissue concentration than an individual with larger body mass in response to a given amount of carotenoid intake (Rock, 1997; Rock & Swendseid, 1993). The conversion of provitamin A carotenoids to vitamin A is very well-regulated, so hypercarotenemia does not cause hypervitaminosis A and these two conditions are unrelated.

Results from several clinical studies and case series reports suggest that abnormal vitamin status may occur in up to one-third of AN patients (Castro et al., 2004; Langan & Farrell, 1985; Phillipp et al., 1988; Rock & Vasantharajan, 1995). In most instances, the observed abnormal levels of indicators represent suboptimal status rather than frank clinical deficiencies. As noted, static measures of many of the vitamins and minerals that have been examined in these studies may not represent overall stores, are influenced by nondietary factors, or reflect recent meals (or low recent intakes). In one study, average erythrocyte folate concentrations in adolescent patients with AN did indicate low reserves of this vitamin (Castro et al., 2004), and this level increased but remained lower than optimal after weight restoration to achieve a BMI of at least 17.5 kg/m^2. This finding suggests that restoration of body reserves for some nutrients, especially in the young patient who may have particularly high requirements due to recovery superimposed on needs for growth, may require time after the immediate weight restoration period. In longitudinal studies, the biochemical measures of nutrients have generally been observed to increase as a result of normalized intakes during refeeding and weight restoration (Castro et al., 2003; Rock & Vasantharajan, 1995). Evidence suggests that thyroid hormone abnormalities that result from severe dietary restriction may adversely affect riboflavin status by causing an impaired metabolism of the vitamin to the active coenzyme forms (Capo-chichi et al., 1999). The latter finding is of clinical importance because this suggests that an improvement in energy balance, and thus, overall nutritional status (rather than simply providing the vitamin), may be necessary to correct the problem.

The primary feature of the diets of patients with AN is a deficit of energy intake relative to expenditure. Early studies suggested an average intake of 800–1,200 kcal/day in stable but low-weight patients (Gwirtsman, Kaye, Curtis, & Lyter, 1989; Rock & Curran-Celentano, 1996). However, the diet varies with stage of illness, because greater dietary restriction becomes necessary to promote continued weight loss. Data from a longitudinal study, in which 3-day food records were available for analysis at 2 years and 1 year before the onset of AN and during the first year of the illness, indicate a significantly lower total energy intake (compared to healthy girls) at the 1-year but not the 2-year pre-onset assessment (Affenito, Dohm, Crawford, Daniels, & Striegel-Moore, 2002). During the first year of illness, the girls who had developed AN reported lower total energy and fat intakes compared to the healthy girls (averaging 1,446 vs. 1,823 kcal/day, and 26.7% vs. 31.7% energy from fat, respectively). In AN patients participating in a clinical trial that did not focus on weight restoration, a detailed diet history was collected prior to observing 1 day's intake during hospitalization, and these dietary data were compared with similar data from control subjects (Hadigan et al., 2000). For the patients with AN (but not the control subjects), a strong positive correlation between diet history and observed intakes was observed for energy, macronutrients, and micronutrients. However, the estimated dietary intakes from the diet history were considerably higher than the observed intakes (i.e., averaging 1,602 vs. 1,289 kcal/day for energy), suggesting substantial overreporting of intakes in this patient population.

Additional features of the diets of these patients are individual idiosyncratic patterns, such as avoidance of fat or preference for sweet flavors. Eating patterns, such as eating foods in a particular order or at certain times of the day, are carefully regulated and highly individualized. Prolonged mealtimes, unusually seasoned foods or combinations of foods, or excessive amounts of coffee or low-calorie soft drinks are believed to be a conscious or unconscious strategy to manage hunger as a general response to semistarvation (Rock & Curran-Celentano, 1996). Patients with the binge–purge subtype of AN have episodes of binge eating superimposed on their usual energy-restricted diets.

The issue of estimating energy requirements in these patients is clinically important, because this information should form the basis of the prescribed or goal energy intake to promote weight restoration. Some investigators and clinicians have hypothesized that patients with AN may have increased energy requirements due to psychological stress or other metabolic abnormalities, which would theoretically facilitate weight loss. As recently reviewed (de Zwaan, Aslam, & Mitchell, 2002), current evidence suggests that resting energy expenditure in AN patients who are maintaining a low body weight does not differ from control subjects when expressed as a function of lean body mass. In free-living AN patients maintaining a low body weight, substantially increased levels of physical activity (rather than hypermetabolism per se) explain higher than expected total energy expenditure (Casper, Schoeller, Kushner, Hnilicka, & Gold, 1991). During the refeeding process, resting energy expenditure increases dramatically compared to prediction equations derived from observations of normal subjects who are not eating high-energy diets to promote weight gain (Krahn et al., 1993), presumably as a result of metabolic effects of the refeeding regimen. In clinical practice, this means that higher than expected levels of intake may be necessary to enable progressive weight restoration. In one study, diet-induced thermogenesis in response to a carbohydrate load (but not in response to a fat load) was higher in AN patients than in control subjects (Russell et al., 2001). However, because the relative contribution of this component of energy expenditure is small, the clinical significance of this finding is unknown. Whether there are differential effects of variable macronutrient composition on weight gain in these patients has not been examined in controlled clinical studies. Ideally, the energy requirement of an individual patient with AN should be based on measures of resting energy expenditure with indirect calorimetry, which is a noninvasive and relatively inexpensive technique for measuring this major determinant of the total requirement (Schebendach, 2003).

BULIMIA NERVOSA

By definition, patients with BN do not present with low body weight, as is characteristic of AN; instead, they are usually within the normal range of weight for height. However, frequent and significant weight fluctuations are common in these patients, as is a desire for a body weight that is unrealistically low.

As with patients with AN, micronutrient abnormalities also occur in these patients, in addition to clinical laboratory abnormalities related to neuroendocrine dysfunction associated with dieting behavior, such as hypercholesterolemia (Vize & Coker, 1994). In general, the degree of nutritional compromise and dietary restriction is the most important determinant of risk for these abnormalities. Depending on the nonbinge diet, various degrees of energy imbalance occur in BN, so abnormalities that result from a severe energy deficit are often, but not always observed in these patients. Dehydration and electrolyte abnormalities caused by purging, such as hypokalemia and hypochloremic alkalosis, are common.

The diagnostic criteria for BN focus on the binge eating (and purging) behaviors, but another key characteristic of the dietary pattern in BN is dietary restriction. Numerous studies of the dietary intakes and eating patterns of patients with BN have been conducted, as summarized in a comprehensive review by Guertin (1999). In addition to providing comparative data in the nutritional assessment of these patients, these data inform the research on theoretical models describing etiology and perpetuating factors for this disorder.

A key feature of their dietary intakes is that when not binge eating, patients with BN consume less energy and lower amounts of fat than the general population (Gendall, Sullivan, Joyce, Carter, & Bulik, 1997). For example, the average meal for patients with BN on a nonbinge day in an observational laboratory study provided 242 kcal, compared with 368 kcal in control subjects (Kaye et al., 1992). Specific food choices are based on rules such as good or bad and safe or forbidden, rather than simply on calories per se (Kales, 1990). Thus dietary restriction in the patient with BN is defined by both the quantity of foods consumed and, what is more important, their characteristics (e.g., palatability, attributes, associated cognitions). In one cohort of patients with BN, foods most frequently rated as forbidden included cake, cookies, bread, ice cream, fried foods, and butter, and foods rated as safe included vegetables, fruit, chicken, fish, lean meat, and yogurt (Kales, 1990). This dichotomous approach is reflected in the nutrient composition of intakes during nonbinge meals and episodes compared to binge episodes. In a study based on food records, average intakes during nonbinge episodes (compared to binge episodes) were higher in percent energy from protein (16.4% vs. 11.5%) and lower in percent energy from fat (30.0% vs. 41.6%) and sugar (9.5% vs. 12.4%) (Gendall et al., 1997). This pattern of restriction appears to set the stage for binge eating when the patient perceives an opportunity to purge after the forbidden foods are eaten (Guertin, 1999). Also, this observation supports the theory that restraint plays some role in perpetuating binge eating in this population and provides some rationale for the nutrition intervention. In these patients, the nutrition intervention addresses expanding the allowed foods and increasing meal regularity and amounts consumed, rather than simply focusing on the factors triggering or associated with the binge eating episodes per se.

A number of studies have examined the energy content of binges in this patient population, although some constraints apply when comparing data collected using various methodologies. As noted, factors influencing under- and overestimation of intakes are differentially affected by the method of collecting the dietary data (e.g., food records, laboratory studies). Also, the variable severity of illness of patients studied across the different research settings is also likely to influences the observations. Sometimes a nonbinge meal becomes a binge during the meal, when a self-imposed food rule is violated and the opportunity to purge is evident. Observational studies have consistently found that binges typically average > 1,000 kcal (and > 2,000 kcal in most laboratory-based studies), and that there is large within- and between-subject variability in the amount of food consumed in an episode of binge eating (Guertin, 1999). The amount of food retained despite self-induced vomiting (the most common purging strategy) explains the maintenance of normal body weight despite the baseline restrictive diet and binge eating episodes. Vomiting does not completely prevent the utilization of energy from binge eating. An average retention of approximately 1,200 kcal from binges of various sizes and energy contents was observed in one study (Kaye, Weltzin, Hsu, McConaha, & Bolton, 1993). Laxative use has minimal effect on absorption of energy-producing macronutrients (Bo-Linn, Santa Ana, Morawski, & Fordtran, 1983), although that strategy promotes transient weight loss due to dehydration.

A small subgroup (< 10%) of patients with BN report that binge eating preceded dieting, and these patients appear to more closely resemble individuals with binge eating disorder (discussed later in this chapter), with consistently higher body weights (Haiman & Devlin, 1999). Intakes of this subgroup have not been compared with intakes of the majority of this patient population, in whom weight concerns, dieting behavior, and efforts to control body weight generally preceded the establishment of the binge eating pattern.

Several investigations of energy expenditure, especially resting energy expenditure (the major component of total energy expenditure), have been conducted in patients with BN, but the results have been inconsistent (de Zwaan et al., 2002). Notably, it has been suggested that active involvement in binge–purge behavior may influence resting energy expenditure in these patients, with abstinence associated with either decreased or increased energy requirements. Thus the patient's clinical and behavioral status should be considered in the interpretation of these measures, especially if they are conducted and examined over time.

Discontinuing purging behaviors is an important aspect of intervention for most patients with BN, and this usually results in rebound fluid retention and associated weight gain. Regular eating and activity patterns, plus consistent daily intakes of carbohydrate, sodium, and energy, will eventually result in normal sodium (and fluid) balance. Severe dietary sodium restriction may actually aggravate the problem of fluid retention in these patients, because counterregulatory mechanisms, such as increased aldosterone secretion, are highly responsive due to periods of dehydration and electrolyte depletion.

BINGE EATING DISORDER

Binge eating disorder (BED) is currently included in the category of eating disorder not otherwise specified (EDNOS), as a subgroup with provisional criteria in the fourth edition of the *Diagnostic and Statistical Manual of Mental Disorders* (American Psychiatric Association, 1994). EDNOS is a rather heterogeneous diagnostic category that is applicable for individuals who have clinically significant eating disorders but who fail to meet all the diagnostic criteria for the main eating disorders, AN or BN. The diagnostic criteria for binge eating disorder are considered provisional rather than definite because less evidence has been accumulated to define the disorder and to differentiate it from other eating disorders and psychiatric problems as a distinct condition. In studies that attempt to characterize the nutritional status and dietary patterns of this population, criteria applied to distinguish subjects with this disorder from comparison groups are somewhat variable, which affects the interpretation of results and explains some of the inconsistencies.

Patients with BED do not use purging behaviors on a regular basis, yet they binge eat binge regularly, so they are typically obese (Marcus,

1993). These patients are usually identified when they seek treatment for their obesity, rather than presenting for treatment of an eating disorder. A consistent finding in studies comparing patients with BED with non-binge-eating obese patients is that the binge eating patients are typically more obese (Marcus, 1993; Telch, Agras, & Rossiter, 1988). In contrast with patients with BN, a pattern of dieting behavior preceding the establishment of the binge eating pattern does not appear to be characteristic of a clear majority of these patients. Approximately 50% of patients with BED report that they started binge eating before they started dieting or trying to lose weight (Mussell et al., 1995; Wilson, Nonas, & Rosenblum, 1993).

Because these patients are typically obese, clinical laboratory data relating to nutritional status usually reflect the metabolic changes associated with obesity (Expert Panel on the Identification, Evaluation, and Treatment of Overweight in Adults, 1998). These laboratory findings include increased fasting triacylglycerol concentration, reduced high-density lipoprotein cholesterol concentration, increased fasting and postprandial insulin concentrations, and elevated postprandial glucose concentration (with the latter factors suggesting insulin resistance and glucose intolerance). Comorbidities such as hypertension, type 2 diabetes mellitus, atherosclerotic cardiovascular disease, sleep apnea, and nonalcoholic steatohepatitis are relatively common in obese individuals and should be considered in their nutritional assessment (Aronne, 2002; Kushner & Roth, 2003; Yousseff & McCullough, 2002).

The dietary intakes and eating patterns of patients with BED have been examined in several studies. Knowledge of how their intakes and patterns may differ from other groups, especially nonbinge-eating obese patients or patients with BN, would be useful in the refinement of diagnostic criteria. In general, studies have shown that patients with BED ingest significantly more energy on binge days (but not on nonbinge days) when compared with non-binge-eating obese individuals matched for age and BMI (Raymond, Neumeyer, Warren, Lee, & Peterson, 2003; Yanovski et al., 1992). A proportionately higher intake of fat on binge days (vs. nonbinge days) in this population also has been observed in laboratory studies and comparative studies based on random multiple dietary recalls (Raymond et al., 2003; Yanovski et al., 1992). A comparison of dietary data based on food records did not reveal differences between intakes on binge days and nonbinge days in a sample of patients with this disorder (Reeves et al., 2001).

Also, patients with BED may have a characteristic pattern of intake that differs from non-binge-eating obese individuals, with less food being consumed during the midday and more food being consumed in the evening on binge days (Raymond et al., 2003). This pattern suggests an attempt to restrict intake earlier in the day, with subsequently greater likelihood of binge eating, and might provide insight into the refinement of strategies for meal planning and nutrition intervention for this patient population. Results from one comparison of the quantity and quality of intakes during binge eating in patients with BED or BN suggested similar levels of energy but differential distribution of calories, with more fat and less carbohydrate consumed by the former group of patients (Fitzgibbon & Blackman, 2000).

SUMMARY

Nutritional status is often profoundly affected by the cognitions and behaviors characteristic of eating disorders, due to the effects on body weight and dietary intakes. The metabolic and physiological consequences of suboptimal intakes, abnormal nutritional status, and eating patterns serve to perpetuate these disorders. Nutritional assessment involves collecting and evaluating anthropometric measurements (e.g., height, weight), relevant clinical laboratory data, biochemical indicators of nutritional status, estimates of dietary intakes, and data on eating patterns. Although the collection and interpretation of data that go into the nutritional assessment can be challenging, using a multifaceted approach improves the likelihood of accurate diagnosis and the development of an appropriate intervention.

REFERENCES

Affenito, S. G., Dohm, F. A., Crawford, P. B., Daniels, S. R., & Striegel-Moore, R. H. (2002). Macronutrient intake in anorexia nervosa: The National Heart, Lung, and Blood Institute Growth and Health Study. *Journal of Pediatrics, 141*, 701–705.

American Psychiatric Association. (1994). *Diagnostic and statistical manual of mental disorders* (4th ed.). Washington, DC: Author.

Aronne, L. J. (2002). Classification of obesity and assessment of obesity-related health risks. *Obesity Research, 10*(Suppl.), 105S–115S.

Becker, A. E., Grinspoon, S. K., Kubanski, A., & Herzog, D. B. (1999). Eating disorders. *New England Journal of Medicine, 340*, 1092–1098.

Black, A. E., & Cole, T. J. (2001). Biased over- or under-reporting is characteristic of individuals whether over time or by different assessment methods. *Journal of the American Dietetic Association, 101*, 70–80.

Bo-Linn, G. W., Santa Ana, C. A., Morawski, S. G., & Fordtran, J. S. (1983). Purging and calorie absorption in bulimic patients and normal women. *Annals of Internal Medicine*, 99, 14–17.

Capo-chichi, C. D., Gueant, J. L., Lefebvre, E., Bennani, N., Lorentz, E., Vidailhet, C., et al. (1999). Riboflavin and riboflavin-derived cofactors in adolescent girls with anorexia nervosa. *American Journal of Clinical Nutrition*, 69, 672–678.

Caregaro, L., Favaro, A., Santonastaso, P., Alberino, F., Di Pascoli, L., Nardi, M., Favaro, S., & Gatta, A. (2001). Insulin-like growth factor 1 (IGF-1), a nutritional marker in patients with eating disorders. *Clinical Nutrition*, 20, 251–257.

Casper, R. C., Schoeller, D. A., Kushner, R., Hnilicka, J., & Gold, S. T. (1991). Total daily energy expenditure and activity level in anorexia nervosa. *American Journal of Clinical Nutrition*, 53, 1143–1150.

Castro, J., Deulofeu, R., Gila, A., Puig, J., & Toro, J. (2004). Persistence of nutritional deficiencies after short-term weight recovery in adolescents with anorexia nervosa. *International Journal of Eating Disorders*, 35, 169–178.

Curtin, F., Morabia, A., Pichard, C., & Slosman, D. O. (1997). Body mass index compared to dual-energy X-ray absorptiometry: Evidence for a spectrum bias. *Journal of Clinical Epidemiology*, 50, 837–843.

de Zwaan, M., Aslam, Z., & Mitchell, J. E. (2002). Research on energy expenditure in individuals with eating disorders: A review. *International Journal of Eating Disorders*, 31, 361–369.

Dietz, W. H., & Bellizzi, M. C. (1999). Introduction: The use of body mass index to assess obesity in children. *American Journal of Clinical Nutrition*, 70(Suppl.), 123S–125S.

Expert Panel on the Identification, Evaluation, and Treatment of Overweight in Adults. (1998). Clinical guidelines on the identification, evaluation, and treatment of overweight and obesity in adults: Executive Summary. *American Journal of Clinical Nutrition*, 68, 899–917.

Fairburn, C. G., & Beglin, S. J. (1990). Studies of the epidemiology of bulimia nervosa. *American Journal of Psychiatry*, 147, 401–408.

Fitzgibbon, M. L., & Blackman, L. R. (2000). Binge eating disorder and bulimia nervosa: Differences in the quality and quantity of binge eating episodes. *International Journal of Eating Disorders*, 27, 238–243.

Food and Nutrition Board, Institute of Medicine. (1997). *Dietary reference intakes for calcium, phosphorus, magnesium, vitamin D, and fluoride*. Washington, DC: National Academy Press.

Food and Nutrition Board, Institute of Medicine. (1998). *Dietary reference intakes for thiamin, riboflavin, niacin, vitamin B6, folate, vitamin B12, pantothenic acid, biotin, and choline*. Washington, DC: National Academy Press.

Food and Nutrition Board, Institute of Medicine. (2000). *Dietary reference intakes for vitamin C, vitamin E, selenium, and carotenoids*. Washington, DC: National Academy Press.

Food and Nutrition Board, Institute of Medicine. (2001). *Dietary reference intakes for vitamin A, vitamin K, arsenic, boron, chromium, copper, iodine, iron, manganese, molybdenum, nickel, silicon, vanadium, and zinc*. Washington, DC: National Academy Press.

Gendall, K. A., Sullivan, P. E., Joyce, P. R., Carter, F. A., & Bulik, C. M. (1997). The nutrient intake of women with bulimia nervosa. *International Journal of Eating Disorders, 21*, 115–127.

Gold, P. W., Gwirtsman, H., Avgerinos, P. C., Neiman, L. K., Gallucci, W. T., Kaye, W., et al. (1986). Abnormal hypothalamic-pituitary-adrenal function in anorexia nervosa. *New England Journal of Medicine, 314*, 1335–1342.

Grinspoon, S., Thomas, L., Miller, K., Pitts, S., Herzog, D., & Klibanski, A. (2001). Changes in regional fat redistribution and the effects of estrogen during spontaneous weight gain in women with anorexia nervosa. *American Journal of Clinical Nutrition, 73*, 865–869.

Guertin, T. L. (1999). Eating behavior of bulimics, self-identified binge eaters, and non-eating-disordered individuals: What differentiates these populations? *Clinical Psychology Review, 19*, 1–23.

Gwirtsman, H. E., Kaye, W. H., Curtis, S. R., & Lyter, L. M. (1989). Energy intake and dietary macronutrient content in women with anorexia nervosa and volunteers. *Journal of the American Dietetic Association, 89*, 54–57.

Habicht, J. P., & Pelletier, D. L. (1990). The importance of context in choosing nutritional indicators. *Journal of Nutrition, 120*(Suppl.), 1519–1524.

Hadigan, C. M., Anderson, E. J., Miller, K. K., Hubbard, J. L., Herzog, D. B., Klibanski, A., & Grinspoon, S. K. (1999). Assessment of macronutrient and micronutrient intake in women with anorexia nervosa. *International Journal of Eating Disorders, 28*, 284–292.

Haiman, C., & Devlin, M. J. (1999). Binge eating before the onset of dieting: A distinct subgroup of bulimia nervosa. *International Journal of Eating Disorders, 25*, 151–157.

Horner, N. K., Patterson, R. E., Neuhouser, M. L., Lampe, J. W., Beresford, S. A., & Prentice, R. L. (2002). Participant characteristics associated with errors in self-reported energy intake from the Women's Health Initiative food-frequency questionnaire. *American Journal of Clinical Nutrition, 76*, 766–773.

Jernstrom, H., Deal, C., Wilkin, F., Chu, W., Tao, Y., Majeed, N., et al. (2001). Genetic and nongenetic factors associated with variations of plasma levels of insulin-like growth factor-I and insulin-like growth factor-binding protein-3 in healthy premenopausal women. *Cancer Epidemiology, Biomarkers, & Prevention, 10*, 377–384.

Jonnalagadda, S. S., Mitchell, D. C., Smiciklas-Wright, H., Meaker, K. B., Van Heel, N., Karmally, W., et al. (2000). Accuracy of energy intake data estimated by a multiple-pass, 24-hour dietary recall technique. *Journal of the American Dietetic Association, 100*, 303–308.

Kales, E. F. (1990). Macronutrient analysis of binge eating in bulimia. *Physiology and Behavior, 48*, 837–840.

Kaye, W. H., Weltzin, T. E., Hsu, L. K., McConaha, C. W., & Bolton, B. (1993). Amount of calories retained after binge eating and vomiting. *American Journal of Psychiatry, 150*, 969–971.

Kaye, W. H., Weltzin, T. E., McKee, M., McConaha, C., Hansen, D., & Hsu, L. K. G. (1992). Laboratory assessment of feeding behavior in bulimia and healthy women: Methods for developing a human-feeding laboratory. *American Journal of Clinical Nutrition, 55*, 372–380.

Kerruish, K. P., O'Connor, J., Humphries, I. R. J., Kohn, M. R., Clarke, S. D., Briody,

J. N., et al. (2002). Body composition in adolescents with anorexia nervosa. *American Journal of Clinical Nutrition, 75*, 31–37.

Krahn, D. D., Rock, C. L., Dechert, R. E., Nairn, K. K., & Hasse, S. A. (1993). Changes in resting energy expenditure in anorexia nervosa patients during refeeding. *Journal of the American Dietetic Association*, 93, 434–438.

Kushner, R. F., & Roth, J. L. (2003). Assessment of the obese patient. *Endocrinology and Metabolism Clinics of North America, 32*, 915–933.

Langan, S. M., & Farrell, P. M. (1985). Vitamin E, vitamin A and essential fatty acid status of patients hospitalized for anorexia nervosa. *American Journal of Clinical Nutrition, 41*, 1054–1060.

Marcus, M. D. (1993). Binge eating in obesity. In C. G. Fairburn & G. T. Wilson (Eds.), *Binge eating: Nature, assessment, and treatment* (pp. 77–96). New York: Guilford Press.

Mazzone, A., & Dal Canton, A. (2002). Hypercarotenemia. *New England Journal of Medicine, 346*, 821.

Mussell, M. P., Mitchell, J. E., Weller, C. L., Raymond, N. C., Crow, S. F., & Crosby, R. D. (1995). Onset of binge eating, dieting, obesity, and mood disorders among subjects seeking treatment for binge eating disorder. *International Journal of Eating Disorders, 17*, 395–410.

Nelson, M., Black, A. E., Morris, J. A., & Cole, T. J. (1989). Between- and within-subject variation in nutrient intake from infancy to old age: Estimating the number of days required to rank dietary intakes with desired precision. *American Journal of Clinical Nutrition, 50*, 155–167.

Novotny, J. A., Rumpler, W. V., Riddick, H., Hebert, J. R., Rhodes, D., Judd, J. T., et al. (2003). Personality characteristics as predictors of underreporting of energy intake on 24-hour dietary recall interviews. *Journal of the American Dietetic Association, 103*, 1146–1151.

Phillipp, E., Pirke, K. M., Seidl, M., Tuschl, R. J., Fichter, M. M., Eckert, M., et al. (1988). Vitamin status in patients with anorexia nervosa and bulimia nervosa. *International Journal of Eating Disorders*, 8, 209–218.

Probst, M., Goris, M., Vandereycken, W., & Van Coppenolle, H. (2001). Body composition of anorexia nervosa patients assessed by underwater weighing and skinfold-thickness measurements before and after weight gain. *American Journal of Clinical Nutrition, 73*, 190–197.

Raymond, N. C., Neumeyer, B., Warren, C. S., Lee, S. S., & Peterson, C. B. (2003). Energy intake patterns in obese women with binge eating disorder. *Obesity Research, 11*, 869–879.

Rebro, S. M., Patterson, R. E., Kristal, A. R., & Cheney, C. L. (1998). The effect of keeping food records on eating patterns. *Journal of the American Dietetic Association*, 98, 1163–1165.

Reeves, R. S., McPherson, R. S., Nichaman, M. Z., Harrist, R. B., Roreyt, J. P., & Goodrick, G. K. (2001). Nutrient intake of obese female binge eaters. *Journal of the American Dietetic Association, 101*, 209–215.

Rock, C. L. (1997). Carotenoids: Biology and treatment. *Pharmacology & Therapeutics, 75*, 185–197.

Rock, C. L., & Curran-Celentano, J. (1996). Nutritional management of eating disorders. *Psychiatry Clinics of North America, 19*, 701–713.

Rock, C. L., Gorenflo, D. W., Drewnowski, A., & Demitrack, M. A. (1996). Nutritional characteristics, eating pathology, and hormonal status in young women. *American Journal of Clinical Nutrition, 64,* 566–571.

Rock, C. L., & Swendseid, M. E. (1993). Plasma carotenoid levels in anorexia nervosa and in obese patients. *Methods in Enzymology, 214,* 116–123.

Rock, C. L., & Vasantharajan, S. (1995). Vitamin status of eating disorder patients: Relationship to clinical indices and effect of treatment. *International Journal of Eating Disorders, 18,* 257–262.

Russell, J., Baur, L. A., Beumont, P. J. V., Byrnes, S., Gross, G., Touyz, S., et al. (2001). Altered energy metabolism in anorexia nervosa. *Psychoneuroendocrinology, 26,* 51–63.

Russell, J. D., Mira, M., Allen, B. J., Stewart, P. M., Vizzard, J., Arthur, B., et al. (1994). Protein repletion and treatment in anorexia nervosa. *American Journal of Clinical Nutrition, 59,* 98–102.

Schebendach, J. (2003). The use of indirect calorimetry in the clinical management of adolescents with nutritional disorders. *Adolescent Medicine, 14,* 77–85.

Taren, D. L., Tobar, M., Hill, A., Howell, W., Shisslak, C., Bell, I., et al. (1999). The association of energy intake bias with psychological scores of women. *European Journal of Clinical Nutrition, 53,* 570–578.

Telch, C. F., Agras, W. S., & Rossiter, E. M. (1988). Binge eating increases with increasing adiposity. *International Journal of Eating Disorders, 7,* 115–119.

Vaisman, N., Corey, M., Rossi, M. F., Goldberg, E., & Pencharz, P. (1988). Changes in body composition during refeeding of patients with anorexia nervosa. *Journal of Pediatrics, 113,* 925–929.

Vize, C. M., & Coker, S. (1994). Hypercholesterolemia in bulimia nervosa. *International Journal of Eating Disorders, 15,* 293–295.

Wentz, E., Mellstrom, D., Gillberg, C., Sundh, V., Gillberg, I. C., & Rastam, M. (2003). Bone density 11 years after anorexia nervosa onset in a controlled study of 39 cases. *International Journal of Eating Disorders, 34,* 314–318.

Wilson, G. T., Nonas, C. A., & Rosenblum, G. D. (1993). Assessment of binge-eating in obese patients. *International Journal of Eating Disorders, 13,* 25–33.

Yanovski, J. A. (2001). Pediatric obesity. *Reviews in Endocrine & Metabolic Disorders, 2,* 371–383.

Yanovski, S. Z., Leet, M., Yanovski, J. A., Flood, M., Gold, P. W., Kissileff, H. R., et al. (1992). Food selection and intake of obese women with binge-eating disorder. *American Journal of Clinical Nutrition, 56,* 975–980.

Youssef, W. I., & McCullough, A. J. (2002). Steatohepatitis in obese individuals. *Best Practice and Research Clinical Gastroenterology, 16,* 733–747.

CHAPTER 9

Family Assessment

Daniel le Grange

The association between family functioning and disordered eating has received a great deal of attention over the years. In their assessment of these families, clinicians and researchers alike have alluded to the impact, mostly negative, that family interactions might have on the development of eating disorders. Consequently, a belief has developed that the families of patients with anorexia nervosa (AN) and bulimia nervosa (BN) have qualities specific to these disorders (Dare, 1985; Humphrey, 1992; Yager, 1982).

Examining family issues in eating disorders is not new. The earliest descriptions of AN, in both the English and the French literature, ascribed a crucial role to the way in which the patient and family interact and the way in which this interaction influences the development and the outcome of the illness. In 1873 William Gull described the family of AN patients as the "worst attendants" in their care, while Charcot went a step further in 1889 when he described the influence of the parents as "particularly pernicious." Also in 1873, Charles Lasègue had a more positive view of family influences when he said that one should always consider the "preoccupations of the parents side by side with that of the patient."

These disparate views of the family are reflected in a continuing divide today. One side sees the family as pathological or a hindrance that should either be excluded from treatment (e.g., "parentectomy") or included, but with the "pathological family interactions" modified through treatment (Minuchin, Rosman, & Baker, 1978; Palazzoli, 1974). The other side regards it as premature to refer to a "typical" eating disorder family (Dare, Le Grange, Eisler, & Rutherford, 1994); instead, those holding this view believe that the family should be seen as a resource and part of the solution (Eisler, Dare, Hodes, Russell, & Le Grange, 2000).

To review the developments around the assessment of families of patients with an eating disorder, the first part of this chapter provides a theoretical background that defines the eating disorder family. Most of this research is based on AN as very little is known about BN families. The various family assessment methods, both self-report and observer ratings, are discussed in the second part. The chapter then turns to the assessment of the family of the adolescent patient in particular, then briefly deals with the limited information that focuses on the assessment of adult patients with eating disorders and their families. In the fifth part of this chapter, we review the differences between AN and BN before drawing some conclusions and presenting directions for future study.

THEORETICAL BACKGROUND

One of the first systematic investigations that addressed the question of what goes on in families where a child suffers from an eating disorder was conducted by Bruch and Touraine (1940). Mainly concerned with childhood obesity, Bruch and Touraine postulated a disturbance in the psychological climate in these families. Later on, but primarily working with the individual patient with AN, Bruch (1970, 1971, 1973, 1977) emphasized the importance of the family's influence on this illness by stating that treatment was likely to fail unless the family was involved. Palazzoli demonstrated this change from an individual to a family focus to an even greater degree. Following considerable case experience in the use of individual treatment for AN in the 1960s, she developed a sense of dissatisfaction with this approach and began to insist upon the participation of the whole family in the treatment of AN (Palazzoli, 1970, 1974, 1978).

Consequently, family dynamics have for many decades now been implicated in the development and perpetuation of eating disorders. In particular, the efforts of the Philadelphia Child Guidance Clinic demonstrated that the anorexic child is not merely a passive recipient of "noxious environmental influences" but part of a process of feedback between the individual and other family members that serves to perpetuate the illness. By the end of the 1970s, extensive descriptions of the nature of the relationships within AN families were established.

DESCRIPTION OF AN FAMILIES

Despite considerable variation in characteristics among families whose offspring have an eating disorder, there have been numerous attempts to define the typical AN family. For instance, Bruch (1970) commented that these families find it hard to acknowledge any disharmony and members deny all problems other than the patient's eating difficulties. Therefore, the family has little reason to quarrel and functions with a façade of normalcy. However, it was the descriptions of the family constellation in AN provided by Palazzoli (1970, 1974) and Minuchin and his colleagues (Minuchin et al., 1975, 1978) that focused attention on certain "unique qualities" of AN families.

Palazzoli described the systemic–strategic family model for eating disorders. She was one of the first to propose that AN developed from a whole pattern of family events over at least three generations; the illness maintains and at the same time is maintained by a circular sequence of transactions in the family. Approaching the problem in this way led her to the discovery that certain family components were quite directly and specifically related to AN and that these components could be modified by family therapy (Palazzoli, 1970). Her team observed the interaction of AN families during treatment and generated six interactional hypotheses: (1) relationships tend to be rigidly defined, and the only "escape" for the adolescent is the anorexic symptoms; (2) the family is leaderless; (3) no coalitions are accepted; (4) no responsibility is taken for personal behavior, which makes the AN acceptable because the patient "cannot help it," "she's ill," and all decisions are for someone else's "good"; (5) blame is shifted around and although the mothers tend to overly blame themselves, they describe their behavior as an expression of their devotion to their children; (6) the child is used as a go-between for parents and has no remaining energy to become independent. This is referred to as "three-way matrimony" and any attempt by the child to escape is met by concerted parental opposition (Palazzoli, Boscolo, Cecehin, & Prata, 1980).

Arguably, the most elegant and thorough description of the observed characteristics of families with an adolescent who has an eating disorder is that provided by Minuchin and his colleagues (1975, 1978). Formulating a family systems model, these authors described three necessary conditions for the development and maintenance of severe psychosomatic problems in families: (1) a certain kind of family organization that encourages somatization, (2) involvement of the child in parental conflict, and (3) a physiological vulnerability. Family interactional patterns may trigger the onset or hamper the psychophysiological processes, or both.

The resultant anorexic symptoms are postulated to function as a regulator of family transactions and therefore serve as a homeostatic mechanism. According to Minuchin, the family with an anorexic child is typified by four structural transactional characteristics: (1) enmeshment, which is identified by a high degree of responsiveness in the family, and interaction is characterized by a high degree of involvement with one another, e.g., family members might answer for one another; (2) overprotectiveness, which is manifested by both children and parents being very concerned for one another not limited to the identified patient or to the illness; (3) rigidity, which expresses itself as a need to maintain the status quo and makes periods of change and growth very difficult; and (4) lack of conflict resolution, which expresses itself in either by maintaining a low threshold for conflict, which implies that no explicit negotiation of differences are allowed, or by poor resolution of conflict, with the result that problems remain unresolved, or when they resurface, the family's avoidance circuits are swiftly activated.

The second strand of this family model pertains to the physiological vulnerability of the child. The third condition postulates that the ill child plays an important role in the conflict-avoidance behavior, which at the same time serves as an important reinforcement for the symptom. This aspect is important because, unlike the four preceding characteristics, which imply a causal link, this family characteristic implies the operation of a more complex and multidimensional process. Three patterns of involvement are related to psychosomatic illness. The first two patterns, triangulation and parent–child coalition, are characterized by a split in the spouse dyad and the child is openly pressed to ally with one parent against the other. The third pattern, detouring, implies a united spouse subsystem. The parents submerge their conflicts and, in a united way, either blame or protect their sick child, as the child's illness is defined as the only problem. Minuchin and his colleagues (1978) argue that changing these typical family characteristics is a prerequisite for successful treatment.

Since these earlier descriptions of the AN family, well-matched clinical portrayals of such families to those of the Philadelphia group have been provided (Dare, 1983; Eisler, 1988; Humphrey, 1989; Sargent, Liebman, & Sliver, 1985; White, 1983; Yager & Strober, 1985). For instance, Yager and Strober (1985) summarized descriptions of the stereotypic AN family as upper-middle-class and achievement-oriented, with family members being very weight- and exercise-conscious. A great deal of emphasis is placed on the external appearances of these families, and their members often display a congenial exterior. These authors concede, however, that the ability of the available hypotheses to offer explanations is very limited, given the heterogeneity of the syndrome of AN. They echo the sentiments of many authorities in the field of eating disorders (Morgan & Russell, 1975) when they said that patients show great diversity with respect to many factors, such as age at onset, ego strength, psychosexual development, and a variety of other clinical features.

While Minuchin has provided an eloquent description of the typical psychosomatic family, efforts to verify his description of these families failed to provide evidence in support of this typology (e.g., Burbeck, 1979; Kagan & Squires, 1985), and criticized it for its methodological weaknesses (Kramer, 1988; Wood & Talman, 1983). Kog, Vandereycken, and Vertommen (1985a, 1985b) also could not support Minuchin's claim that all anorexic families can be described by specific interactional characteristics. They argue that Minuchin's description leaves little room for variation within these families, overemphasizes pathology, and is characterized by a considerable degree of overlap between the various constructs, (e.g., overprotectiveness vs. enmeshment). They added that a generalized family typology is not possible as neither the age of the patient nor the symptomatology seem to be connected to a particular type of family functioning (Kog, Vertommen, & Vandereycken, 1987). These authors concede that eating disorder families could be typified as consistently less inclined to discuss disagreements between family members and also more rigid in their family organization when compared with normal controls. They also noted that anorexic and bulimic families differ in important ways and it would therefore be misleading to speak of a typical eating disorder family (Kog & Vandereycken, 1989). Even before Kog and her colleagues' (1987) rebuke of the limitations of accepting a simplified definition of eating disorder families, several other authors (e.g., Crisp, Harding, & McGuinness, 1974; Grigg, Friesen, & Sheppy, 1989; Kalucy, Crisp, & Harding, 1977) have noted that family psychopathology is diverse and that few universal familial patterns can be recognized in eating disorder families.

In a comprehensive evaluation of Minuchin's psychosomatic model, Dare and his colleagues (1994) used Expressed Emotion (Vaughn & Leff, 1976) and the Family Adaptability and Cohesion Evaluation Scales (Olson, Sprenkle, & Russell, 1979) to validate this typology of the AN family. These authors concluded that their data show some agreement with Minuchin's and other clinical accounts of family makeup in AN, but they go on to say that their findings amplify rather than simply confirm or contradict them.

ASSESSMENT METHODS

Since the early work of authorities such as Bruch, Palazzoli, and Minuchin, a body of evidence has emerged that suggests the quality of family relationships might be closely related to the development, maintenance, and treatment response in patients with eating disorders. In the work to improve understanding of these processes, several assessment measures have been developed to tap into the family life of patients with eating disorders. The next section of this chapter presents the most prominent and frequently used methods of assessing these families. Assessments are typically conducted for research and clinical purposes, mostly using self-report and observer-based methods.

Self-Report Measures

Using self-report to assess patients and their families has obvious disadvantages: for example, an exclusive reliance on the subject's understanding of the assessment method and assessment procedures accompanied by little, if any, clarification by the assessor, social desirability, defensiveness, response bias, and a dependence on retrospective recall of information or perception, which can be inaccurate. On the other hand, an obvious advantage of self-report measures is that they are often time-efficient ways of tapping into the subject's personal or emotional life experiences. At least two comprehensive and well-known models of family functioning with concomitant self-report measures have been developed: the Circumplex Model of Marital and Family Systems (Olson et al., 1979) and the McMaster Model of Family Functioning (Epstein, Baldwin, & Bishop, 1983). Both these models have been validated by a comparison of symptomatic with nonsymptomatic families. The McMaster model appears to be superior in terms of its ability and sensitivity to identify clinical families, as well as in the correspondence between clinical and self-ratings (Fristad, 1989; Miller et al., 1994).

The Circumplex model relies on the Family Adaptability and Cohesion Evaluations Scales (FACES-III; Olson et al., 1979; Olson, Portner, & Lavee, 1985) to arrive at a description of family functioning. The FACES is 20-item self-report questionnaire developed by Olson and his colleagues for the study of family process using family systems theory as its framework. FACES aims to assess the family members' experience of their lives together along two dimensions: family cohesion (closeness or distance) and family adaptability (rigidity or flexibility). "Cohesion" is the degree of bonding that family members have with one another, and "adaptability" indicates the ability of a family to change its power structures, rules, and roles in response to stressful situations. The FACES-III assesses family functioning both as it is perceived (how family members currently view their family), and as it is idealized (how they would like it to be). In addition, the level of each individual's dissatisfaction with family life can be calculated by comparing the perceived-ideal discrepancies for every member of the family: the greater the discrepancy, the greater the dissatisfaction. The theoretical model that underlies this questionnaire is that of a Circumplex model in which disordered families are characterized as deviating from normal functioning. Normality is thought to lie in a balanced style with neither too much nor too little closeness and neither too much nor too little adherence to rules (Olson et al., 1979).

Several studies have used FACES to assess family characteristics of patients with eating disorders (Dare et al., 1994; Le Grange, Eisler, Dare, & Russell, 1992; Wallin & Kronvall, 2002) and found that AN families, in terms of their FACES-*Ideal* scores, express a desire for a closer organization. Also, AN families have ideals for a pattern of family life that is characterized by a low level of hierarchy and a low level of domination by rules. No information about BN families or comparisons with non–eating disorder groups are available.

The McMaster model of family functioning is best assessed using the Family Assessment Device (FAD; Epstein et al., 1983). The FAD is a 60-item self-report scale (although the original had 53 items) designed to assess family functioning along seven dimensions and is based on the McMaster Model of Family Functioning (Epstein, Bishop, & Levin, 1978). Six of these scales reflect dimensions of family functioning as outlined in the McMaster Model of Family Functioning: Problem Solving, Communication, Roles, Affective Responsiveness, Affective Involvement, and Behavior Control. The seventh dimension, General Functioning, assesses overall health or pathology. The psychometric properties of the FAD have been established with scale reliabilities favorable and generally supportive of the factor structure of this measure (Epstein et al., 1983; Kabacoff, Miller, Bishop, Epstein, & Keitner, 1990; Miller, Epstein, Bishop, & Keitner, 1985; Sawyer, Sarris, Cross, & Kalucy, 1988).

The FAD is perhaps the assessment tool most frequently used to assess the perception of family functioning by patients with eating disorders and their parents (e.g., Emanuelli et al., 2004; Gowers & North, 1999; McDermott, Batik, Roberts, & Gibbon, 2002; McGrane & Carr, 2002; North, Gowers, & Byram, 1995; Steiger, Liquornik, Chapman, & Hussain, 1991; Waller, Slade, & Calam, 1990). Waller and his colleagues (1990) have found the FAD helpful as a measure of pathology in the families of both AN and BN women. These authors conclude that it was the patients, as opposed to their parents, who had the most realistic perceptions of their families' interactional styles.

McDermott et al. (2002) had 80 children and adolescents with AN, BN, and eating disorder not otherwise specified (EDNOS) and their parents complete the FAD. They found no differences in scores for the parents and their children. "Community norms" were established by examining the Western Australian Child Health Survey. Subjects in this study scored significantly higher in family dysfunction than the norm. There was no significant difference in the total scores of family functioning for all eating disorder groups, although the BN groups reported difficulty in the areas of family activity planning, decision making, and family interactions when compared to the other eating disorder groups.

Also using the FAD, McGrane and Carr (2002) evaluated the relationship between perceived family dysfunction, parental psychological problems, and the risk for eating disorders in young women. Twenty-seven subjects regarded as at risk for an eating disorder and 27 control subjects completed the FAD, among other measures. The at-risk group scored significantly higher than the control group for family problems in general functioning as well as roles, affective responsiveness, and problem solving. The at-risk group also reported their mothers to have more problems with depression, anxiety, and sensitivity (among other areas) than the control group, and their fathers to have more anger, hostility, and depression.

Several other self-report measures of family life have been used in eating disorder studies, albeit less frequently; here are brief summaries. The Family Assessment Measure (FAM; Skinner, Steinhauer, & Santa-Barbara, 1983) is a self-report measure of family functioning; the Family Environment Scale (FES; Moos, 1974) assesses the family social environment as perceived by one or more family member; the Family Dynamics Survey (FDS; Berren & Shisslak, 1980) assesses family characteristics such as closeness, emotional support, independence, and quality of communication, and the Family Relations Scale (FARS; Cederblad & Hook, 1992) is a 46-item self-rating questionnaire including five factors: attribution, interest, isolation, chaos, and cohesion. For additional information on the use of self-report measures with patients with eating disorders, please see Chapter 6.

Observational Methods

Observational methods have the obvious advantage that they are investigator-based and therefore more reliable than self-report measures in arriving at an accurate description of family interactional characteristics. Observational assessments usually require observer training, and administering the assessments can be cumbersome and time-consuming. Consequently, fewer of these methods have been employed in the assessment of patients with eating disorders compared to self-report measures. Although only a few studies are available, the most frequently used observer assessment method for the families of patients with eating disorders has been expressed emotion (EE; Vaughn & Leff, 1976). EE is a measure of relatives' attitudes toward an ill member of the family. EE is traditionally rated from an audiotaped semistructured interview with a single relative of the afflicted offspring, the Camberwell Family Interview (CFI; Brown, Birley, & Wing, 1972; Vaughn & Leff, 1985). The shorter version of the original interview still lasts about two hours, making it quite cumbersome in either clinical or research settings. This interview is mainly concerned with the relative's account of the patient's behaviors and his or her reaction to these behaviors.

Rating EE along its subscales is as time-consuming as the interview, taking on average between one and two additional hours. EE is measured on five principal subscales: Critical Comments (CC), Hostility (H), Emotional Overinvolvement (EOI), Warmth (W), and Positive Remarks (PR). Ratings are based on the content, tone, and expression of voice using audiotapes of the CFI. CC and PR are both based on frequency counts, while H, EOI, and W are global ratings. An extended period of training is required to become a reliable EE rater. EE has been demonstrated as an excellent predictor of relapse in patients with schizophrenia and depression (Leff & Vaughn, 1989), and some studies have also used the CFI to assess the emotional climate in AN families (Szmukler, Eisler, Russell, & Dare, 1985; Van Furth et al., 1996). Reliability for EE is always established by way of a two-week training course with a trained EE rater. Agreement between the trainee and the established EE rater is established at a mean correlation coefficient of at least .80 for all five EE subscales. A kappa coefficient for interrater agreement in terms of high-EE versus low-EE should be achieved at a level no lower than .70. Construct validity of EE has primarily been established through a series of studies of direct family interaction experiments and interaction coding (e.g., Affective Style [AS]; Doane, West, Goldstein, Rodnick, & Jones, 1981; "Kategoriensystem fur Partnerschaftliche Interaktion" [KPI]; Hahlweg et al., 1984). Taken together, these studies have demonstrated that high EE on CFI or AS are highly predictive of negative interaction between parents and their offspring.

EE can be assessed in a variety of ways and several attempts have been made to simplify the rating process to make it more applicable for research and everyday clinical practice. Most economical is Magana and coworkers' (1986) adaptation of the Five-Minute Speech Sample (FMSS), which was originally developed by Gottschalk and Gleser (1969). Coding EE with the FMSS allows for the evaluation of both tone and content of the speech sample. Both criticism and emotional overinvolvement are assessed, with high CC, EOI, or both yielding the final high/low EE designation. Van Furth, Van Strien, Van Son, and Van Engeland (1993) have employed the FMSS in a sample of adolescents with AN and reported that this instrument takes 7 minutes to administer and 15 minutes to rate. If the FMSS can replace the CFI to rate EE, its use and applicability will be greatly extended. Similar to the few prior studies of EE among patients with eating disorders (Le Grange, Eisler, Dare, & Hodes, 1992; Szmukler, Berkowitz, Eisler, Leff, & Dare, 1987), Van Furth and his colleagues (1993) also found levels of CC to be low among the relatives of young patients with AN. These authors conclude that the FMSS and CFI-EE ratings showed only a modest degree of overlap, and state that at this time it would be premature to replace the CFI with the FMSS to rate EE in AN families.

Another alternative to the CFI is whole-family interviews. At least three studies (Eisler et al., 2000; Le Grange, Eisler, Dare, & Russell, 1992; Wallin & Kronvall, 2002) used the Standardized Clinical Family Interview (SCFI; Kinston & Loader, 1984), which is faster to administer than the CFI. The SCFI is a semistructured interview typically used for families without an ill offspring. This interview covers several aspects of family life and all family members are encouraged to participate in these discussions. As mentioned, the most important advantage of using the SCFI is that it is less time-consuming than the conventional CFI. For instance, one interview allows ratings from both parents as well as other family members. As Hodes, Dare, Dodge, and Eisler (1999) also point out, such a method could help to bridge the therapy–research gap in showing how responses to clinically relevant questions can be linked to research findings. These authors compared the assessment of EE using the SCFI and found moderate correlation between the SCFI and the CFI for critical comments, emotional overinvolvement, and warmth. These authors concluded that the SCFI is useful in assessing EE.

The *family meal*, where people bring their own meals to the therapist's office, allows the therapist to assess the family's regular habits around eating (who cooks, who dishes up, etc.), and also gives the therapist an opportunity to support the parents in their efforts to have their AN offspring eat one bite more than he or she had intended. This procedure, first described by Minuchin's group (Minuchin et al., 1978; Rosman, Minuchin, & Liebman, 1975a, 1975b), has served as a focus for treatment in AN and has been described as an important tool to assess the way in which the family organizes itself around the dilemma of getting their adolescent offspring to eat more than he or she is prepared to (Dare, 1983; Jaffa, Honig, Farmer, & Dilley, 2002; Le Grange, Eisler, Dare, & Russell, 1992; Lock, Le Grange, Agras, & Dare, 2001; Scholz & Asen, 2001). An alternative model of the family meal in AN, which is seen as stress-inducing, has been presented for BN. Franko (1993) describes a group treatment program for patients with BN in which repeated exposure to the feared event (i.e., eating) is supposed to reduce anxiety. Szmukler, Berkowitz, Eigler, Leff, and Dare (1987) performed EE ratings in two separate settings comparing the conventional CFI with videotaped family meal interviews for patients with AN. These videotaped sessions were relatively unstructured. During the first half of the session the therapist asked the family to discuss, in a neutral way, what their typical eating behaviors are like. The patient's eating disorder is also discussed, also in a simple "fact-finding" manner. In the second part of the session, the therapist exerted pressure on the parents to convince their offspring to eat more than he or she was prepared to in order to examine the way in which the family responded to this stress-inducing intervention. Comparison of ratings for the family meal and the CFI showed a high correlation for critical comments. These authors concluded that rating EE in this way provides new possibilities for the study of families, especially in clinical settings. When EE is applied in a family setting, it may prove fruitful in terms of generating hypotheses about how particular families function and EE may therefore be a much-needed reliable basis to describe patterns of family interaction.

Taken together, these various studies have all demonstrated that the levels of criticism, when compared to families with a schizophrenic offspring, emerged as exceptionally low in the relatives of youngsters with eating disorders (Le Grange, Eisler, Dare, & Hodes, 1992; Szmukler, Eisler, Russell, & Dare, 1985; Szmukler, Berkowitz, et al., 1987; Van Furth et al., 1993, 1996). Less is known about levels of EE in the families whose offspring have BN. However, these authors have suggested that, given the nature of the bulimic syndrome, it is likely that BN families tend to be more critical of their offspring (Dare et al., 1994; Szmukler et al., 1987). EE has proved a fruitful avenue of inquiry and is worthy of further investigation into the climate of all eating disorder families (Hodes & Le Grange, 1993).

Additional Observational Methods

Other than EE, some additional observational methods have been implemented in the assessment of eating disorder families. The family task, which was developed by Minuchin et al. (1978), involves engaging a family along a series of interactive tasks that they administer and carry out by themselves. This technique enables the researcher to study the family in a quasi-natural setting without having to interview the family. This method consists of five questions that are prerecorded on tape; the family can start and stop the recording by themselves, arrange or seat themselves as they wish, and answer the questions only if they wish. The five tasks that are put to the family in succession are (1) to make up a menu together, (2) to discuss a family argument, (3) to describe what pleases and displeases them about other family members, (4) to make up stories about family pictures, and (5) to put together a color forms design (which is to be copied from a design provided to the family) (Minuchin et al., 1978).

All discussions and transactions are videotaped and then scored by an independent rater. These recordings are scored along the four primary structural characteristics of the typical psychosomatic family, i.e., enmeshment, overprotectiveness, low tolerance for conflict, and rigidity. Minuchin and his colleagues (1978) admitted that operationalizing these constructs was a challenge and that more work in this area was needed. However, they concluded that psychosomatic families (families whose offspring had anorexia, asthma, or diabetes) can be characterized by these distinct interactional patterns and that these families are descriptively and clinically in tone different from normal control families.

Developed by Luborsky and Crits-Christoph (1990), the Core Conflictual Relationship Theme method (CCRT) is an assessment measure that has been used frequently in the field of quantifying relationship diagnoses. Similar to a clinical assessment, the CCRT is a standardized analysis of interpersonal narratives that aims to identify patterns in the responses of one person in interaction with relevant others. CCRT aims to identify patterns that tend to be repeated, and these narratives are referred to as "relationship episodes" that are then examined for three components: the subject's wish, need, or intention, which in turn leads to responses of those around the subject (others), and consequently leads to a return response by the subject (self). Narrative material is typically collected either from therapy records or from so-called relationship anecdotes paradigm interviews (Luborsky, 1990).

Using the CCRT, Benninghoven and colleagues (Bennighoven, Schneider, Strack, Reich, & Cierpa, 2003) evaluated family dynamics among three adult groups of patients with eating disorders: 17 with BN, 18 clinical controls, and 20 nonclinical controls. The CCRT was applied to narrative material for all three groups. While the results showed no differences between the two clinical groups, these groups exhibited lower levels of cohesion and expressiveness and more conflict compared to the normal controls.

CLINICAL ASSESSMENT: THE FAMILY INTERVIEW AND THE ADOLESCENT PATIENT

Outside the research-oriented assessments of eating disorder families, as outlined thus far, several clinical accounts of the assessment of these families have been developed over the years (e.g., Andersen, 1985; Dare & Szmukler, 1991; Jack, 2001; Lask & Bryant-Waugh, 1993; Lock et al., 2001; Minuchin et al., 1978; Woodside & Shekter-Wolfson, 1991). As one would expect, given the prominence of Minuchin's original work in describing the makeup of psychosomatic families, his account of the family diagnostic interview is perhaps best known (Minuchin et al., 1978). Whereas the family task, briefly discussed earlier, provides the opportunity to study the four structural characteristics of the "anorexic family," the family diagnostic interview was designed to evaluate the index patient's involvement in parental conflict, as well as to assess the physiological effects of that parental conflict may have on the adolescent's illness. A key characteristic of this interview was to expose any conflict between parents based on issues that are idiosyncratic to that family. The therapist's role in this scenario is to exacerbate the conflict between the parents to a level above their usual threshold before introducing the adolescent patient into the situation. The resultant interaction between the parents and their offspring (triadic interaction) is then evaluated for both its psychological content and its physiological consequences (Minuchin et al., 1978). This process, it is argued, allows the interviewer to study the adolescent's physiological responses to the emotional arousal brought about by being triangulated in the parental conflict. Unlike the family task, the process of triadic interaction does not permit the inclusion of other family members.

Andersen (1985) provided his own outline of essential information to survey for a clinical assessment of the family. This includes an evaluation of the following six family characteristics: (1) interactional patterns (the affective climate of the family), (2) flexibility (the ease with which family members move from one role to another), (3) sensitivity (the balance of concern or support shown and the ability to provide age-appropriate independence), (4) support available to the family and significant stressors (the availability of supportive friends or relatives and work and financial situations and stressors), (5) performance of developmentally appropriate tasks (age-appropriate rights and responsibilities), and (6) family knowledge of the illness (the family's knowledge of the patient's behavior and their general knowledge of eating disorders).

Finally, Dare and Szmukler (1991) advocate an "observing team" to scrutinize, modify, and further develop the therapist's responses to the family. This observing team observes the therapist and the family from behind a one-way mirror. At certain times throughout the assessment, the therapist may join the team behind the mirror to confer regarding their collective assessment of the family thus reducing the risk that the assessor (the therapist) might unconsciously "fit in" with family patterns, that is, fail to remain an objective observer. Should this happen, the therapist and the family will be less effective at resolving the adolescent's eating disorder.

THE FAMILY OF THE ADULT PATIENT

Many patients with eating disorders are adolescents who live with their families of origin. Adult patients, on the other hand, present with a greater variety of living arrangements, that is, living alone or with their family of origin, or, increasingly, in marriages or committed relationships of their own (Woodside, Lackstrom, & Shekter-Wolfson, 2000). However, compared to adolescents and their families, much less information is available about the assessment of the family of an adult patient (e.g., Van den Broucke & Vandereycken, 1989a, 1989b; Woodside & Shekter-Wolfson, 1991). Adult patients living with their families of origin tend to receive scant attention. By contrast, there is a relatively rich literature on the marriages of adult patients (e.g., Van den Broucke, Vandereycken, & Vertommen, 1995; Van Den Broucke, Vandereycken, & Norre, 1997; Woodside, Shekter-Wolfson, Brandes, & Lackstrom, 1993). These reports describe troubled relationships sometimes caused by the eating disorder and sometimes where the eating disorder seems to have arisen in an attempt to bring some resolution to the troubled relationship. Most of the reports paint a bleak picture of these marital relationships and offer a poor prognosis in the event of the resolution of the eating disorder (Woodside, Lackstrom & Shekter-Wolfson, 2000).

Most studies have presented a mixed picture of marital relationships for adult patients with eating disorders. Van den Broucke, Vandereycken, and Vertommen (1995), using an observational measure of communication patterns, found that eating disorder couples, compared to maritally distressed and maritally nondistressed couples, had generally better communication and more self-disclosure compared to the other two groups. A group from Japan (Kiriike, Nagata, Matsunaga, Tobitan, & Nishiura, 1996, 1998) reported that marital distress was a significant trigger in more than 70% of cases where the eating disorder onset occurred after the marriage had begun. These findings led Woodside and his colleagues (2000) to look at marital satisfaction and intimacy of couples in which one member has an eating disorder, using the Waring Intimacy Questionnaire (WIQ; Waring & Reddon, 1983). The WIQ is a 90-item true–false questionnaire developed specifically to measure marital intimacy. Woodside and his colleagues administered the WIQ at admission and again at discharge to a group of patients and their spouses who attended a day-hospital program. Self-reported marital dissatisfaction among patients with eating disorders was at least partially alleviated with symptomatic improvement. However, treatment of one member of the couple does not necessarily lead to less marital dissatisfaction in the other member of the couple.

Results from the available studies also present a mixed picture of the quality of the relationships when one member has an eating disorder. This area of inquiry has received little research attention, in part because relatively few AN patients are in committed relationships. However, BN patients are less likely to shy away from such relationships and little, if any, research has looked into the assessment of these new families.

ARE THERE DIFFERENCES BETWEEN ANOREXIA NERVOSA AND BULIMIA NERVOSA?

Although AN and BN have many shared characteristics, these disorders can also be distinguished from each other in several meaningful ways. Therefore, descriptions of the AN family do not necessarily apply to the family with a BN patient. As the preceding part of this chapter has mostly focused on the family with an AN patient, the discussion now turns to what is known about the family with a BN patient. Compared with AN, patients with BN and their families have also received relatively less attention, although some studies have compared perceived family interactions in AN and BN family members with normal control families. Humphrey (1986a), using the FACES, found that bulimic families were consistently more distressed, less involved and supportive, and more isolated, conflictual, understructured, and detached compared to normal controls. Based on her clinical impression of the families, Humphrey states that the bulimic families reflected a pattern of dysregulation and poor modulation of affect and impulses similar to that commonly seen in the bulimic patient. She also states that these families can become chaotic, impulsive, labile, and more likely to express their hostility and frustration with one another. Bulimics and their parents feel ineffective in regulating painful and dysphoric affect relative to normal controls and the entire family shows deficits in nurturance and empathy, as well as excesses in terms of criticism and neglect, when compared to normal families.

In a similar study of "bulimic–anorexic" versus nondistressed families, Humphrey (1986b) found that the families with an eating disorder patient were more "hostile, detached and chaotic than overprotective and overinvolved" (p. 231), as well as more disturbed in terms of the frequent use of negativistic, complex, and contradictory communications. In yet another study by Humphrey (1986c), patients with either AN or BN were found to be different from "normal young women" in that they viewed their parents as more blaming, rejecting, and neglectful. Ordman and Kirschenbaum (1986) examined the family projections of women with BN compared to normal controls, also using the FACES. They found their results to be inconclusive regarding the hypothesis that BN, like AN, represents a young person's dilemma in separating from an overinvolved family. Based on this hypothesis, these patients should have had high measures on cohesion, but contrary to expectations, the bulimic subjects reported less cohesion.

When the differences between AN and BN families are scrutinized more closely, it appears that bulimics and their parents experience intergenerational boundaries as relatively impenetrable and describe their families as less involved, less supportive, and more distressed and conflictual than the families described by patients with restricting AN (Kog & Vandereycken, 1989). Patients with restricting AN and their parents tend to perceive the family in similar ways, but they experience more difficulties with task accomplishment, role performance, communication, and affective expression than normative controls (Garfinkel et al., 1983). AN families also show less tolerance of conflict or the expression of negative emotional states and show greater cohesiveness, whereas BN patients feel more alienated from their parents. Parents of BN patients also show greater psychiatric morbidity when compared with families of patients with restricting AN (Dare et al., 1994; Goldstein, 1981; Kog & Vandereycken, 1989; Strober & Humphrey, 1987; Van Furth et al., 1996).

Additional disparities between the families with an anorexic child and families with a bulimic child have been noted. For instance, critical comments as assessed with EE seem to be at higher levels for relatives with a bulimic offspring (Dare et al., 1994). This finding is in keeping with those of other researchers who have described BN families as more conflictual than AN families (Dolan, Lieberman, Evans, & Lacey, 1990; Goldstein, 1981; Strober, 1981; Szmukler et al., 1985). Families with an anorexic child also report more warm and positive remarks (Dare et al., 1994), and perceive their families as being closer than is the case of those with a bulimic offspring (Humphrey, 1986a; Kog & Vandereycken, 1989).

Finally, while Minuchin and his colleagues' (1978) psychosomatic model assumes the existence of a pattern that pertains, for example, to diabetic families as well as those containing an anorexic or bulimic patient, it would appear that there might be differences between bulimic and anorexic families. Such a difference would contradict the notion of a universal pattern that applies to all families wherein a child has a psychosomatic problem.

HOW-TO: FAMILY ASSESSMENT FOR PRACTITIONERS

- It is essential that thorough physical and psychological assessments of the adolescent patient have been conducted prior to meeting with the family for the initial assessment.
- It is most helpful if all members of the family who live under the same roof attend the family assessment meeting. This strategy sets out to involve both parents (if it is a two-parent family) from the outset, and it provides information about the patient *and* the family that is otherwise unavailable.

Three main goals are identified for the family assessment meeting:

1. Engage the family.
2. Obtain a history of the eating disorder and how it affects the family.
3. Gain preliminary information about family functioning—coalitions, authority structure, conflicts, and so on.

How should the practitioner go about achieving these goals?

- As in any treatment, the first priority is to establish rapport with the family. Inquire a little about everyone present's life—questions like What work do you do? What grade are you in? Where do you live? Ask how they have learned about coming to the meeting and what their thoughts are about being at the meeting.
- Ask the parents how they see the development of the eating disorder occurring—that is, when they first perceived it to be a problem, what they did to try to help, whether there are other problems such as anxiety or depression, and if they have noticed any other changes in their child's behavior.
- Finally, try to get a general picture of the patient's emotional and physical development. In addition, ask about any possible family problems in general, and also about family weight and shape concerns in particular.

SUMMARY

Although there are widely discrepant views about the characteristics of families containing a patient with an eating disorder, and notwithstanding the possible influence of other variables, few authorities today would question the role of family factors in the pathogenesis and maintenance of eating disorders. Indeed, a family approach to the study of eating disorders has become widely influential in the United States, Europe, and elsewhere. In this approach, the family is viewed as a self-regulating system and is characterized by certain transactional patterns, redundancies in communication, and subsystems in which affiliation depends on age, role, and other factors. From this perspective, the patient's symptoms are thought to be evoked, supported, and reinforced by certain parental characteristics and family transactions. When the individual's symptoms are placed in the context of the family, "the development crisis of adolescents is as much a crisis for the whole family as it is for the individual" (Eisler, Dare, & Szmukler, 1988, p. 101).

A wide variety of assessment methods for families of patients with eating disorders are available, which does make it somewhat difficult to compare results among studies. Findings are often discrepant and it is not surprising that some authors find scant evidence for psychopathology among the parents or the families of patients with eating disorders. Moreover, the literature that is concerned with the assessment of the families of patients with eating disorders has several shortcomings. For instance, the assumption that the same influences are at work at different stages of these syndromes—onset, process, and recovery—is unwarranted. Furthermore, much of the work in this field is impressionistic and speculative. Thus one can at best conclude that the individuals in these families exhibit a wide range of personalities and dynamics and that the difficulties experienced by these families in relationships can be seen as universal problems in the developmental crises of many troubled families.

Further research might be useful in several areas. The most obvious is perhaps the direction of causality; a prospective study would be helpful to establish whether family interaction leads to eating disorders or vice versa. Also, some of the pathological family attributes were not specific to eating disorders. For instance, Benninghoven et al. (2003) found that the eating disorder group and non-eating disorder clinical group in their study shared many similarities compared to a normal control group. In other instances, researchers found no differences between the eating disorder and normal control groups (e.g., Solomon, Klump, McGue, Iacono, & Elkins, 2003). And finally, in some studies parents tended to perceive their families in a more favorable light compared to the opinion of their offspring, regardless whether or not their child had an eating disorder (Dancyger, Fornari, Scionti, Wisotsky, & Mandel, 2003; Davis, Blackmore, & Kirsh, 2002).

The pressing question remains whether elevated scores on measures of psychopathology in families whose child has an eating disorder precede the onset of the eating disorder, or if these family issues are the consequence of the eating disorder. The methodological design in most of the studies that were discussed in this chapter hampers our ability to answer this question with any certainty. A large number of the studies are cross-sectional. The most obvious shortcoming therefore is that it is difficult to establish whether family issues contribute to eating disorders, whether eating disorders contribute to family dysfunction, or whether a common factor contributes to both. Second, in many studies the role of family dysfunction was ascertained by retrospective recall and self-report, further undermining the certainty of the role family dynamics plays in eating disorders. Third, several studies did not include a control group, which removes any certainty whether these family issues are unique to eating disorder families.

Another area for future inquiry is the need to eliminate the conceptual uncertainties that plague many of the studies presented here, for example, the considerable overlap between constructs of Minuchin's typology of the eating disorder family and the vagueness of revised alternatives (e.g., Kog, Vandereycken, & Vertommen, 1985a; Kog, Vertommen, & Vandereycken, 1987; Kog & Vandereycken, 1989). It is also uncertain to what extent general theoretical models of family functioning such as the Circumplex Model of Marital and Family Systems (Olson et al., 1979) or the McMaster Model of Family Functioning (Epstein et al., 1983) correspond with the psychosomatic model (cf. Dare et al., 1994). The feasibility of evaluating the family interactional characteristics as defined by the psychosomatic model with self-report measures needs to be considered, as well as the correspondence between self-report and observer ratings. Only then will we be in a position to conclude more reliably about typical family features in eating disorders—if any typical features exist.

This chapter confirms the need for more concise conceptual descriptions and theoretical syntheses of family interactional concepts. This would facilitate comparison between diagnostic groups and the investigation of the relationship between family process and symptomatology. One way to resolve this dilemma, as suggested by Waller and his colleagues (1990), is a common model of family functioning, which ought to make it easier to relate family interaction to abnormal eating. It must be stressed, however, that even if a discernable pattern of family organization is identified in AN or BN families, this pattern does not establish a connection between such findings and the etiology of the patient's condition—a consistent family structure does not necessarily identify a causal factor in the development of an eating disorder.

REFERENCES

Andersen, A. E. (1985). Family therapy and marital therapy of anorexia nervosa and bulimia. In A. E. Anderson (Ed.), *Practical comprehensive treatment of anorexia and bulimia* (pp. 135–148). Baltimore: Johns Hopkins University Press.

Benninghoven, D., Schneider, H., Strack, M., Reich, G., & Cierpka, M. (2003). Family representations in relationship episodes of patients with a diagnosis of bulimia nervosa. *Psychiatry and Psychotherapy, 76,* 323–336.

Berren, M., & Shisslak, C. M. (1980). *Family dynamics survey.* Tucson: Southern Arizona Mental Health Center and Arizona Health Sciences Center.

Brown, G. W., Birley, J. L. T., & Wing, J. K. (1972). Influence of family life on the course of schizophrenic disorders: A replication. *British Journal of Psychiatry, 121*, 241–258.

Bruch, H. (1970). Family background in eating disorders. In E. J. Anthony & C. Koupernick (Eds.), *The child in his family* (pp. 285–309). New York: Wiley-Interscience.

Bruch, H. (1971). Family transactions in eating disorders. *Comprehensive Psychiatry, 12*, 238–248.

Bruch, H. (1973). Eating disorders: Obesity, anorexia nervosa and the person within. New York: Basic Books.

Bruch, H. (1977). Psychological antecedents of anorexia nervosa. In R. A. Vigersky (Ed.), *Anorexia nervosa* (pp. 1–10). New York: Raven Press.

Bruch, H., & Touraine, G. (1940). Obesity in childhood: V. The family frame of obese children. *Psychosomatic Medicine, 11*, 141–206.

Burbeck, T. W. (1979). An empirical investigation of the psychosomatogenic model. *Journal of Psychosomatic Research, 23*, 327–337.

Cederblad, M., & Hook, B. (1992). *FARS—Family relation scale research on families and children*. Lund, UK: Department of Child and Youth Psychiatry, University of Lund.

Crisp, A. H., Harding, B., & McGuinness, B. (1974). Anorexia nervosa: Psychoneurotic characteristics of parents: Relationship to prognosis. *Journal of Psychosomatic Research, 18*, 167–173.

Dancyger, I., Fornari, V., Scionti, L., Wisotsky, W., & Mandel, F. S. (2003). Do parents see their families as dysfunctional as their daughters with eating disorders do? *International Journal of Eating Disorders, 34*, 8.

Dare, C. (1983). Family therapy for families containing an anorectic youngster. In *Understanding anorexia nervosa and bulimia*. Report of the Fourth Ross Conference on Medical Research (pp. 28–37). Columbus, OH: Ross Laboratories.

Dare, C. (1985). The family therapy of anorexia nervosa. *Journal of Psychiatric Research, 19*, 435–443.

Dare, C., Le Grange, D., Eisler, I., & Rutherford, J. (1994). Redefining the psychosomatic family: Family process of 26 eating disorders families. *International Journal of Eating Disorders, 16*, 211–226.

Dare, C., & Szmukler, G. (1991). Family therapy of early-onset, short-history anorexia nervosa. In D. B. Woodside & L. Shekter-Wolfson (Eds.), *Family approaches in treatment of eating disorders* (pp. 23–48). Washington, DC: American Psychiatric Press.

Davis, C., Blackmore, E., & Kirsh, C. (2002, May). *Family physical activity patterns in hospitalized females with anorexia nervosa: A case control study*. Paper presented at the 2002 AED International Conference on Eating Disorders, Boston, MA.

Doane, J. A., West, K. L., Goldstein, M. J., Rodnick, E. H., & Jones, J. E. (1981). Parental communication deviance and affective style: Predictors of subsequent schizophrenia spectrum disorders in vulnerable adolescents. *Archives of General Psychiatry, 38*, 679–685.

Dolan, B. M., Lieberman, S., Evans, C., & Lacey, J. H. (1990). Family features associated with normal body weight bulimia. *International Journal of Eating Disorders, 9*, 639–647.

Eisler, I. (1988). Family therapy approaches to anorexia. In D. Scott (Ed.), *Anorexia and bulimia nervosa: Practical approaches* (pp. 95–107). London: Croom Helm.

Eisler, I., Dare, C., & Szmukler, G. I. (1988). What's happened to family interaction research? An historical account and a family systems viewpoint. *Journal of Marital and Family Therapy, 14*, 45–65.

Eisler, I., Dare, C., Hodes, M., Russell, G. F. M., Dodge, E., & Le Grange, D. (2000). Family therapy for adolescent anorexia nervosa: The results of a controlled comparison of two family interventions. *Journal of Child Psychology and Psychiatry and Allied Disciplines, 41*, 727–736.

Emanuelli, F., Ostuzzi, R., Cuzzolaro, M., Baggio, F., Lask, B., & Waller, G. (2004). Family functioning in adolescent anorexia nervosa: A comparison of family members' perceptions. *Eating and Weight Disorders, 9*, 1–6.

Epstein, N. B., Baldwin, L. M., & Bishop, D. S. (1983). The McMaster family assessment device. *Journal of Marital and Family Therapy, 9*, 171–180.

Epstein, N. B., Bishop, D. S., & Levin, S. (1978). The McMaster model of family functioning. *Journal of Marriage and Family Counseling, 4*, 19–31.

Franko, D. (1993). The use of a group meal in the brief group therapy of bulimia nervosa. *International Journal of Group Psychotherapy, 43*, 237–242.

Fristad, M. (1989). A comparison of the McMaster and circumplex family assessment instruments. *Journal of Marital and Family Therapy, 15*, 259–269.

Garfinkel, P. E., Garner, D. M., Rose, J., Darby, P. L. Brandes, J. S., O'Hanlon, J., et al. (1983). A comparison of characteristics in the families of patients with anorexia nervosa and normal controls. *Psychological Medicine, 13*, 821–828.

Goldstein, M. J. (1981). Family factors associated with schizophrenia and anorexia nervosa. *Journal of Youth and Adolescence, 10*, 385–405.

Gottschalk, L. A., & Gleser, G. C. (1969). *The measurement of psychological states through analysis of verbal behavior.* Berkeley: University of California Press.

Gowers, S., & North, C. (1999). Difficulties in family functioning and adolescent anorexia nervosa. *British Journal of Psychiatry, 174*, 63–66.

Grigg, D. N., Friesen, J. D., & Sheppy, M. I. (1989). Family patterns associated with anorexia nervosa. *Journal of Marital and Family Therapy, 15*, 29–42.

Gull, W. W. (1873). *Anorexia nervosa (Apepsia Hysterica, Anorexia Hysterica)*. Paper presented at The Trans. Clinical Society (London), 7, 22–28.

Hahlweg, K., Reisner, L., Kohli, G., Vollmer, M., Schindler, L., & Revenstorf, D. (1984). Development and validation of a new system to analyze interpersonal communication (KPI: Kategoriensystem fur Partnerschaftliche Interaktion [Category System for Partners Interaction]). In K. Hahlweg & N. S. Jacobson (Eds.), *Marital interaction: Analysis and modification* (pp. 182–198). New York: Guilford Press.

Hodes, M., Dare, C., Dodge, E., & Eisler, I. (1999). The assessment of expressed emotion in a standardized family interview. *Journal of Child Psychology and Psychiatry, 40*, 617–625.

Hodes, M., & Le Grange, D. (1993). Expressed Emotion in the investigation of eating disorders: A review. *International Journal of Eating Disorders, 13*, 279–288.

Humphrey, L. L. (1986a). Family dynamics in bulimia. In S. C. Feinstein (Ed.), *Ado-*

lescent psychiatry: Development and clinical studies (pp. 315–334). Chicago: University of Chicago Press.

Humphrey, L. L. (1986b). Family relations in bulimic–anorexic and non-distressed families. *International Journal of Eating Disorders, 5*, 223–232.

Humphrey, L. L. (1986c). Structural analysis of parent–child relationships in eating disorders. *Journal of Abnormal Psychology, 95*, 395–402.

Humphrey, L. L. (1989). Observed family interactions among subtypes of eating disorders using structural analysis of social behavior. *Journal of Consulting and Clinical Psychology, 57*, 205–214.

Humphrey, L. L. (1992). Family relations. In K. A. Halmi (Ed.), *Psychobiology and treatment of anorexia nervosa* (pp. 263–286). Washington, DC: American Psychiatric Press.

Jack, S. (2001). Working with families. In J. E. Mitchell (Ed.), *The outpatient treatment of eating disorders: A guide for therapists, dietitians, and physicians* (pp. 187–215). Minneapolis: University of Minnesota Press.

Jaffa, T., Honig, P., Farmer, S., & Dilley, J. (2002). Family meals in the treatment of adolescent anorexia nervosa. *European Eating Disorders Review, 10*, 199–207.

Kabacoff, R., Miller, I., Bishop, D., Epstein, N., & Keitner, G. (1990). A psychometric study of the McMaster family assessment device in psychiatric, medical, and nonclinical samples. *Journal of Family Psychology, 3*, 431–439.

Kagan, D., & Squires, R. (1985). Family characteristics of 105 patients with bulimia. *American Journal of Psychiatry, 142*, 1321–1324.

Kalucy, R. S., Crisp, A. H., & Harding, B. (1977). A study of 56 families with anorexia nervosa. *British Journal of Psychiatry, 50*, 381–395.

Kinston, W., & Loader, P. (1984). Eliciting whole-family interaction with a standardized clinical interview. *Journal of Family Therapy, 6*, 347–363.

Kiriike, N., Nagata, T., Matsunaga, H., Tobitan, W., & Nishiura, T. (1996). Married patients with eating disorders in Japan. *Acta Psychiatrica Scandinavia, 94*, 428–432.

Kiriike, N., Nagata, T., Matsunaga, H., Tobitan, W., & Nishiura, T. (1998). Single and married patients with eating disorders. *Psychiatry and Clinical Neuroscience, 52*, 306–308.

Kog, E., & Vandereycken, W. (1989). Family interaction in eating disorder patients and normal controls. *International Journal of Eating Disorders, 8*, 11–23.

Kog, E., Vandereycken, W., & Vertommen, H. (1985a). Towards a verification of the psychosomatic family model: A pilot study of ten families with an anorexia/bulimia nervosa patient. *International Journal of Eating Disorders, 4*, 525–538.

Kog, E., Vandereycken, W., & Vertommen, H. (1985b). The psychosomatic family model: A critical analysis of family interaction concepts. *Journal of Family Therapy, 7*, 31–44.

Kog, E., Vertommen, H., & Vandereycken, W. (1987). Minuchin's psychosomatic family model revised: A concept-validation study using a multitrait-multimethod approach. *Family Process, 26*, 235–253.

Kramer, S. (1988). Family structure and functional relationships in eating disorders. In B. J. Blinder (Ed.), *Modern concepts of the eating disorders: Research, diagnosis treatment*. New York: Spectrum.

Lasègue, E. C. (1964). De l'anorexie hysterique. In R. M. Kaufman & M. Heiman (Eds.), *Evolution of psychosomatic concepts. Anorexia nervosa: A paradigm* (pp. 384–403). New York: International Universities Press. (Original work published 1873)

Lask, B., & Bryant-Waugh, R. (1993). *Childhood onset anorexia nervosa and related eating disorders*. Hove, UK: Redwood Press.

Le Grange, D., Eisler, I., Dare, C., & Hodes, M. (1992). Family criticism and self-starvation: A study of expressed emotion. *Journal of Family Therapy, 14*, 177–192.

Le Grange, D., Eisler, I., Dare, C., & Russell, G. F. M. (1992). Evaluation of family treatments in adolescent anorexia nervosa: A pilot study. *International Journal of Eating Disorders, 12*, 347–357.

Leff, J., & Vaughn, C. E. (1985). The role of maintenance therapy and relatives' expressed emotion in relapse of schizophrenia: A two-year follow-up. *British Journal of Psychiatry, 139*, 102–104.

Lock, J., Le Grange, D., Agras, W. S., & Dare, C. (2001). *Treatment manual for anorexia nervosa: A family-based approach*. New York: Guilford Press.

Luborsky, L. (1990). A guide to the CCRT method. In L. Luborsky & P. Crits-Christoph (Eds.), *Understanding transference: The Core Conflictual Relationship Theme method* (pp. 82–101). New York: Basic Books.

Luborsky, L., & Crits-Christoph, P. (Eds.). (1990). *Understanding transference: The Core Conflictual Relationship Theme method*. New York: Basic Books.

Magana, A. B., Goldstein, M. J., Karno, M., Miklowitz, D. J., Jenkins, J., & Falloon, I. R. H. (1986). A brief method for assessing expressed emotion in relatives of psychiatric patients. *Psychiatry Research, 17*, 203–212.

McDermott, B. N., Batik, M., Roberts, L., & Gibbon, P. (2002). Parent and child report of family functioning in a clinical child and adolescent eating disorders sample. *Australian and New Zealand Journal of Psychiatry, 36*, 509–514.

McGrane, D., & Carr, A. (2002). Young women at risk for eating disorders: Perceived family dysfunction and parental psychological problems. *Family Therapy, 24*, 385–395.

Miller, I., Epstein, N., Bishop, D., & Keitner, G. (1985). The McMaster family assessment device: Reliability and validity. *Journal of Marital and Family Therapy, 11*, 345–356.

Miller, I., Kabacoff, R., Epstein, N., Bishop, D., Keitner, G., Baldwin, L., et al. (1994). The development of a clinical rating scale for the McMaster model of family functioning. *Family Process, 33*, 53–69.

Minuchin, S., Baker, B. L., Rosman, B. L., Liebman, R., Milman, L., & Todd, T. C. (1975). A conceptual model of psychosomatic illness in children: Family organization and family therapy. *Archives of General Psychiatry, 32*, 1031–1038.

Minuchin, S., Rosman, B. L., & Baker, B. L. (1978). *Psychosomatic families: Anorexia nervosa in context*. Cambridge, MA: Harvard University Press.

Moos, R. (1974). *Family environment scale and preliminary manual*. Palo Alto, CA: Consulting Psychologists Press.

Morgan, H. G., & Russell, G. F. M. (1975). Value of family background and clinical features as predictors of long-term outcome in anorexia nervosa: Four-year follow-up study of 41 patients. *Psychological Medicine, 5*, 355–371.

North, C., Gowers, S., & Byram, V. (1995). Family functioning in adolescent anorexia nervosa. *British Journal of Psychiatry, 167*, 673–678.

Olson, D. H., Portner, J., & Lavee, Y. (1985). *FACES III*. Minneapolis: Family Social Science, University of Minnesota.

Olson, D. H., Sprenkle, D. H., & Russell, C. S. (1979). Circumplex Model of marital and family systems: I. Cohesion and Adaptability dimensions, family types and clinical applications. *Family Process, 18*, 3–28.

Ordman, A. M., & Kirschenbaum, D. S. (1986). Bulimia: Assessment of eating, psychological adjustment and family characteristics. *International Journal of Eating Disorders, 5*, 865–878.

Palazzoli, M. (1970). The families of patients with anorexia nervosa. In E. J. Anthony & C. Koupernik (Eds.), *The child in his family* (pp. 319–332). New York: Wiley-Interscience.

Palazzoli, M. (1974). *Self-starvation*. London: Human Context.

Palazzoli, M. (1978). *Self-starvation: From individual to family therapy in the treatment of anorexia nervosa*. Northvale, NJ: Aronson.

Palazzoli, M., Boscolo, L., Cecehin, G., & Prata, G. (1980). *Paradox and counterparadox: A new model in the therapy of the family in schizophrenic transactions*. Northvale, NJ: Aronson.

Rosman, B. L., Minuchin, S., & Liebman, R. (1975a). Input and outcome of family therapy in anorexia nervosa. In J. A. Claghorn (Ed.), *Successful psychotherapy* (pp. 128–139). New York: Brunner/Mazel.

Rosman, B. L., Minuchin, S., & Liebman, R. (1975b). Family lunch session: An introduction to family therapy in anorexia nervosa. *American Journal of Orthopsychiatry, 45*, 846–853.

Sargent, J., Liebman, R., & Silver, M. (1985). Family therapy for anorexia nervosa. In D. M. Garner & P. E. Garfinkel (Eds.), *Handbook of psychotherapy for anorexia nervosa and bulimia* (pp. 257–269). New York: Guilford Press.

Sawyer, M., Sarris, A., Cross, D., & Kalucy, R. (1988). Family assessment device: Reports from mothers, fathers, and adolescents in community and clinic families. *Journal of Marital and Family Therapy, 14*, 287–296.

Scholz, M., & Asen, E. (2001). Multiple family therapy with eating disordered adolescents: Concepts and preliminary results. *European Eating Disorders Review, 9*, 33–42.

Skinner, H. A., Steinhauer, P. D., & Santa-Barbara, J. (1983). The Family Assessment Measure. *Canadian Journal of Community Mental Health, 2*, 91–105.

Solomon, J. W., Klump, K. L., McGue, M., Iacono, W., & Elkins, I. (2003). Parent and child perceptions of the parental relationship in anorexia nervosa. *International Journal of Eating Disorders, 34*, 7–8.

Steiger, H., Liquornik, K., Chapman, J., & Hussain, N. (1991). Personality and family disturbances in eating disorder patients: Comparison of "restricters" and "bingers" to normal controls. *International Journal of Eating Disorders, 10*, 501–512.

Strober, M. (1981). The significance of bulimia in juvenile anorexia nervosa: An exploration of possible etiologic factors. *International Journal of Eating Disorders, 1*, 28–43.

Strober, M., & Humphrey, L. L. (1987). Familial contributions to the etiology and course of anorexia nervosa and bulimia. *Journal of Consulting and Clinical Psychology, 55,* 654–659.

Szmukler, G. I., Berkowitz, R., Eisler, I., Leff, J., & Dare, C. (1987). Expressed emotion in individual and family settings: A comparative study. *British Journal of Psychiatry, 151,* 174–178.

Szmukler, G. I., Eisler, I., Russell, G. F. M., & Dare, C. (1985). Anorexia nervosa, parental expressed emotion and dropping out of treatment. *British Journal of Psychiatry, 147,* 265–271.

Van den Broucke, S., & Vandereycken, W. (1989a). Eating disorders in married patients: Theory and therapy. In W. Vandereycken, E. Kog, & J. Vanderlinden (Eds.), *The family approach to eating disorders* (pp. 333–345). New York: PMA Publishing.

Van den Broucke, S., & Vandereycken, W. (1989b). The marital relationship of patients with an eating disorder: A questionnaire study. *International Journal of Eating Disorders, 8,* 541–556.

Van den Broucke, S., Vandereycken W., & Norre, J. (1997). *Eating disorders and marriage.* New York: Brunner/Mazel.

Van den Broucke, S., Vandereycken W., & Vertommen, H. (1995). Marital communication in eating disorder patients: A controlled observational study. *International Journal of Eating Disorders, 17,* 1–21.

Van Furth, E., Van Strien, D., Martina, L., Van Son, M., Hendrickx, J., & Van Engeland, H. (1996). Expressed emotion and the prediction of outcome in adolescent eating disorders. *International Journal of Eating Disorders, 20,* 19–31.

Van Furth, E., Van Strien, D., Van Son, M., & Van Engeland, H. (1993). The validity of the five-minute speech sample as an index of expressed emotion in parents of eating disorder patients. *Journal of Child Psychology and Psychiatry, 34,* 1253–1260.

Vaughn, C. E., & Leff, J. (1976). The influence of family and social factors on the course of psychiatric illness: A comparison of schizophrenic and depressed neurotic patients. *British Journal of Psychiatry, 129,* 125–137.

Vaughn, C. E., & Leff, J. (1985). The measurement of expressed emotion in the families of psychiatric patients. *British Journal of Social and Clinical Psychology, 15,* 157–165.

Waller, G., Slade, P., & Calam, R. (1990). Who knows best? Family interactions and eating disorders. *British Journal of Psychiatry, 156,* 546–550.

Wallin, U., & Kronvall, P. (2002). Anorexia nervosa in teenagers: Change in family function after family therapy, at 2-year follow-up. *Nordic Journal of Psychiatry, 56,* 363–368.

Waring, E. M., & Reddon, J. (1983). The measurement of intimacy in marriage: The Waring Intimacy Questionnaire. *Journal of Clinical Psychology, 39,* 53–57.

White, M. (1983). Anorexia nervosa: A transgenerational system perspective. *Family Process, 22,* 255–273.

Wood, B., & Talman, M. (1983). Family boundaries in transition: A search for alternatives. *Family Process, 22,* 347–357.

Woodside, D., Lackstrom, J., & Shekter-Wolfson, L. (2000). Marriage in eating disorders: Comparisons between patients and spouses and changes over the course of treatment. *Journal of Psychosomatic Research*, *49*, 165–168.

Woodside, D., & Shekter-Wolfson, L. (1991). Family treatment in the day hospital. In D. B. Woodside & L. Shekter-Wolfson (Eds.), *Family approaches in treatment of eating disorders* (pp. 87–106). Washington, DC: American Psychiatric Press.

Woodside, D. B., Shekter-Wolfson, L., Brandes, J., & Lackstrom, J. B. (1993). *Eating disorders and marriage*. New York: Brunner/Mazel.

Yager, J. (1982). Family issues in the pathogenesis of anorexia nervosa. *Psychosomatic Medicine*, *44*, 43–60.

Yager, J., & Strober, M. (1985). Family aspects of eating disorder. In A. Frances & R. Hales (Eds.), *American psychiatric update IV* (Vol. 4, pp. 481–502). Washington, DC: American Psychiatric Press.

CHAPTER 10

Assessment of Body Image Disturbance

J. Kevin Thompson
Megan Roehrig
Guy Cafri
Leslie J. Heinberg

A large body of research indicates that some form of body image disturbance (BID) affects many adolescents and adults, individuals of both genders, and people from a variety of ethnic backgrounds (Thompson, Heinberg, Altabe, & Tantleff-Dunn, 1999). For eating disorders, DSM-IV-TR lists a BID symptom as one of the necessary criteria for the diagnosis of anorexia nervosa (AN) and bulimia nervosa (BN) (American Psychiatric Association, 2000). Specifically, for AN, one of the DSM criteria is an "intense fear of gaining weight or becoming fat, even though underweight" (p. 589), and for BN, the BID criterion is "self-evaluation is unduly influenced by body shape or weight" (p. 594). Body image issues have also been found to exist in individuals with binge eating disorder (Johnson & Torgrud, 1996). An extensive literature also supports a positive correlation between BID and dieting, eating disturbances, depression, and low self-esteem in both clinical and nonclinical populations (Stice & Agras, 1998; Thompson, 2004a; Thompson et al., 1999).

An evaluation of body image has historically been considered essential to understanding the etiology of eating disorders and for developing optimal interventions. Bruch's (1962) seminal work describing AN asserted that BID was the most important pathognomonic feature of the disorder and that successful treatment of AN "without a corrective change in the body image" (p. 189) was likely to be short-lived. Dozens of studies have demonstrated the link between BID and problematic eating (see Cash & Deagle, 1997, for a meta-analytic review). Prospective and structural modeling studies demonstrate that BID is the most consistent predictor of the onset of eating disturbance (Stice & Hoffman, 2004; van den Berg, Thompson, Brandon, & Coovert, 2002). Further, BID moderates the connection between multiple other risk factors and eating disorders (Thompson, Coovert, Richards, Johnson, & Cattarin, 1995; Veron-Guidry, Williamson, & Netemeyer, 1997). In prospective studies of AN treatment response, BID at the beginning of inpatient treatment predicts greater attrition and less weight gain (e.g., Heinberg, Guarda, & Haug, 2001). Similarly, greater satisfaction with emaciated appearance predicts poorer weight gain and greater likelihood of relapse (Fairburn, Peveler, Jones, Hope, & Doll, 1993). Additional studies suggest that among patients with AN who had successfully completed treatment and had reached goal weight, weight loss relapse was predicted by BID severity at pretreatment, during treatment, and at discharge (Fairburn et al., 1993; Freeman, Thomas, Solyom, & Hunter, 1985).

Body image disturbance is also an important prognostic factor in the treatment of BN. For example, among patients who had ceased all binge eating and vomiting at the end of outpatient therapy, BID at the end of treatment was one of the two best predictors of relapse after 7 months (Freeman et al., 1985). In a sample of female adolescents, Stice and Agras (1998) found that not only did BID predict the onset of binge eating and purging but also that BID predicted the remission of these bulimic behaviors.

In this chapter, we review a variety of facets of BID, with a goal of providing a framework for understanding the theoretical basis for BID and guidelines for the selection of specific measures for its assessment in eating disturbed samples. We begin with an overview of theoretical explanations, followed by a review of specific dimensions of BID and measures designed to assess particular components of BID. Methodological issues and areas for future work in this area conclude our coverage.

THEORETICAL EXPLANATIONS OF BODY IMAGE

The body image literature has exploded over the past several decades, resulting in an excellent and comprehensive handbook (Cash & Pruzinsky,

2002) and the launching of a journal by Elsevier devoted solely to the topic (*Body Image: An International Journal of Research*). Body image disturbance is actually an umbrella term that covers several subdefinitions (dimensions) of the construct. Researchers generally define body image as the internalized representation of one's weight, shape, and appearance. We have previously conceptualized body image disturbance as a multifaceted construct consisting of subjective dissatisfaction, affective qualities, cognitive characteristics, behavioral aspects, and perceptual components (Thompson et al., 1999).

Several theoretical explanations of body image are compelling and helpful in conceptualizing this complex construct. Cash (2002a) has provided one of the broadest models of body image development, which we have adapted and simplified in Figure 10.1. The model includes four organizing principles: (1) socialization by culture; (2) personality characteristics; (3) interpersonal experiences; and (4) activating events and situations. Following sections review these four influences briefly.

Socialization by Culture

Sociocultural etiologies have received enormous attention, primarily because BID appears to be most prevalent in industrialized nations (Tsai, Curbow, & Heinberg, 2003). Western culture's preoccupation with an increasingly thin female ideal encourages widespread dieting behavior in young girls and women (Fairburn, Welch, Doll, Davies, & O'Connor, 1997) and leads to a high level of BID (Heinberg, 1996).

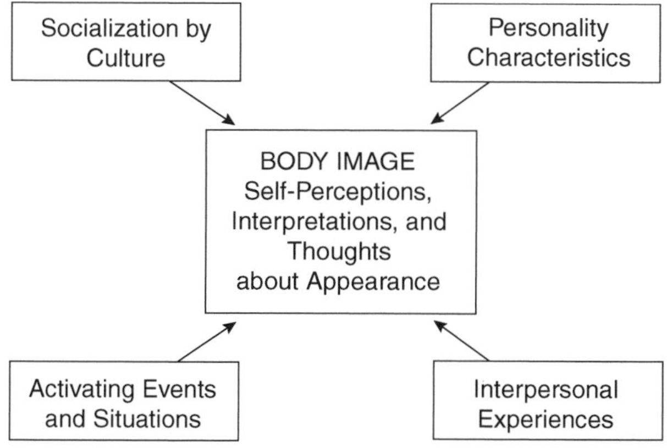

FIGURE 10.1. Theoretical explanations of body image.

Sociocultural Theory

Most researchers agree that sociocultural factors comprise the strongest, most empirically supported influence on the development of body image in Western societies (Thompson et al., 1999). A sociocultural theoretical model asserts that current societal standards for beauty exceedingly stress the importance of thinness (Tiggemann & Pickering, 1996) as well as other unrealistic standards of beauty (Tsai et al., 2003). Sociocultural theory emphasizes that the current societal standard for thinness in women is omnipresent and unfortunately unachievable for the vast majority of women (Thompson & Heinberg, 1999).

Feminist Theory

Striking gender disparities in the prevalence of eating disorders and BID has led to the development of feminist explanations. Some of these feminist theorists build on sociocultural influences, expanding them by explaining that the culture of thinness is a means by which patriarchal society can effectively subjugate women (Gilbert & Thompson, 1996) and that women are far more likely to be have been socialized to equate attractiveness with success (Smolak & Murnen, 2004). Other feminist theorists propose that in order to achieve control in their lives, women define themselves by their body shape and appearance, something that is seemingly under their control (Dworkin, 1988; Szekely, 1989). Finally, feminist theories examine the role of eating disorders as a pathological means of addressing anxieties about female appearance, sexuality, and achievement (Larkin, Rice, & Russell, 1996).

Personality Characteristics

Although the vast majority of individuals are exposed to the thin ideal and cultural expectations of femininity, researchers have begun to examine dispositional variables that may render certain persons at greater risk for sociocultural influence. Two primary moderators have been examined to explain why certain individuals are more sensitive than others to cultural socialization.

Internalization Tendency

An individual difference in the tendency to internalize the thin ideal has received a great deal of attention in recent years (Durkin & Paxton, 2002;

Stice & Shaw, 2002; Thompson & Stice, 2001). Internalization is the endorsement of specific values to the point that they become incorporated into one's own belief system. Thompson and Stice (p. 181) explain internalization as "the extent to which an individual cognitively buys into" societal norms of size and appearance. As a result, individuals are more likely to modify their own behavior in an attempt to meet these ideals. Prevention research has demonstrated that internalization may be a causal risk factor for the onset of eating and shape-related disturbances (Thompson & Stice, 2001). Perhaps most important, researchers have demonstrated that it is possible to modify internalization and that changes in this risk factor appear to be related to changes in levels of body dissatisfaction and eating disturbance (Stice & Hoffman, 2004; Stice, Trost, & Chase, 2003).

Social Comparison Tendency

Another manner in which the cultural ideal of attractiveness is believed to affect an individual's body image is through the process of social comparisons (Heinberg, 1996; Rieves & Cash, 1996). According to social comparison theory, individuals engage in appearance comparisons to determine their status or rank on certain appearance dimensions. Often, these comparisons take the form of "upward comparisons" in which the target for comparison is someone who is more attractive or thinner. Cross-sectional and experimental work has demonstrated the important role appearance-based social comparisons play in predicting body image and eating disturbance (Heinberg & Thompson, 1992; van den Berg et al., 2002; Wertheim, Paxton, & Blaney, 2004).

Interpersonal Experiences

History of Teasing

A wealth of literature supports the notion that teasing, or appearance-related feedback, has a long-term effect on body image (Cattarin & Thompson, 1994; Rieves & Cash, 1996). Teasing history has also been linked to dieting and weight-loss practices (Striegel-Moore, Wilfley, Caldwell, Needham, & Brownell, 1996). Teasing may also disproportionately affect the body image of overweight individuals (Thompson, Coovert, Richards, Cattarin, & Johnson, 1995). Recent work examining the role of mother versus father teasing also suggests that fathers' influence via this method of communication may be more harmful than mothers' (Keery, van den Berg, Boutelle, & Thompson, in press).

Family Attitudes about Appearance

Parents may knowingly or inadvertently help transmit and reinforce sociocultural standards of thinness and appearance to their children (Birch, 1990). Interestingly, these family contextual issues have received far less attention than the more global sociocultural influences. The extant literature suggests that such family attitudes may be communicated via modeling by the parents' own body image and eating behaviors or via the parents' attitudes toward their children's weight, shape, appearance, and diet (Striegel-Moore & Kearney-Cooke, 1994; Thompson et al., 1999). Keery, van den Berg, and Thompson (2004) recently found that family influences explained variance, along with peer and media influences, in the prediction of body image disturbance.

Interpersonal Relationships

Peer influences on girls' and boys' body image have received rather extensive evaluation (e.g., Cafri et al., 2005; Oliver & Thelen, 1996; Smolak, Murnen, & Thompson, in press; Wertheim et al., 2004). These studies indicate that the peer influence may take the form of direct comments (i.e., teasing) or indirect modeling of dietary restriction or body image concerns. Interestingly, very little work has examined the role of a romantic partner in explaining body image issues, although this variable does seem to be an important one (Tantleff-Dunn & Thompson, 1995).

Activating Events and Situations

Pubertal Timing

Researchers have also examined the effect of puberty and pubertal timing on body image development. Generally, early maturation (usually defined by menarche prior to age 11 or self-reported physical maturation earlier than that of peers) is associated with greater body image dissatisfaction (Thompson et al., 1999). More recently, a model that combines early maturation with early dating or academic stress has received support (Levine, Smolak, Moodey, Shuman, & Hessen, 1994; Smolak, Levine, & Gralen, 1993).

Body Mass Index

In general, research strongly supports the commonsense observation that a higher body mass index (BMI) is related to body image dissatisfaction with weight, shape, and appearance (Stice, Mazotti, Krebs, & Martin, 1998; Thompson et al., 1999). However, the relationship between BMI and body image is quite complex, and obese individuals may not necessarily report the expected high levels of BID (Heinberg, Thompson, & Matzon, 2001). Recent research has begun to examine the role of body image dissatisfaction in predicting adherence to weight loss interventions and weight loss maintenance (Cash, 1994; Foster, Wadden, & Vogt, 1997; Heinberg, Haythornthwaite, Rosofsky, McCarron, & Clarke, 2000).

Acute Triggers

Finally, a number of acute triggers have been identified that play an important role in body image development or predict changes in attitudes toward personal appearance. Included in this category are such factors as a history of sexual abuse, sexually inappropriate commentary or sexual harassment, accident or injury, disease (e.g., breast cancer), pregnancy and the postpartum period, aging, and menopause (Cash & Pruzinsky, 2002; Heinberg & Guarda, 2002).

In sum, the area of body image has generated a great deal of work in recent years on the various factors that lead to and maintain disturbances of functioning in this sphere of life. At the same time, researchers have developed a plethora of diverse measures designed to index or assess dimensions of BID. We now turn to an overview of these instruments.

ASSESSMENT OF BODY IMAGE DISTURBANCE

Table 10.1 contains some of the most widely used measures for the assessment of BID. As noted earlier, we have found it useful to subcategorize the measures by the dimension of BID that the scale appears to assess. Only those measures that specifically appear to index an affective, behavioral, perceptual, or cognitive dimension are subgrouped by this designation; others are assigned to the general "subjective dissatisfaction" category. Additionally, Table 10.1 describes three eating disorder interview methods that might also be considered for the measurement of BID because they provide information regarding body image concerns. The Eating Disorder Examination (Fairburn & Cooper, 1993) has been revised multiple times and consists of four subscales, two of which are concerned with BID (Shape Concern and Weight Concern). The Structured Inter-

TABLE 10.1. Measures of Body Image Disturbance

Name of instrument	Authors (year)	Description
Affective measures		
Body Image Quality of Life Inventory	Cash and Fleming (2002)	Assesses the impact of body image on 19 life domains using a 7-point scale ranging from (–3) very negatively to (+3) very positively.
Feelings of Fatness Questionnaire	Roth and Armstrong (1993)	Measures the extent to which females feel "thin–fat" for 61 situations. Has two scales: Troubles (38 items) and Satisfactions (23 items).
Physical Appearance State and Trait Anxiety Scale (PASTAS)	Reed et al. (1991)	Assesses anxiety associated with 16 body sites (eight weight-related, eight non-weight-related); available in trait and state forms.
Situational Inventory of Body Image Dysphoria (SIBID)	Cash (1994)	Forty-eight-item instrument in which adult men and women use a Likert scale to rate how often they experience negative body image emotions in various situations.
Situational Inventory of Body Image Dysphoria—Short Form	Cash (2002b)	Twenty-item shortened form of the SIBID for use in men and women.
Behavioral measures		
Body Checking Questionnaire	Reas, Whisenhunt, and Netemeyer (2002)	Twenty-three-item scale measures body-checking behaviors related to overall appearance, specific body parts, and idiosyncratic checking behaviors in adult females.
Body Image Avoidance Questionnaire	Rosen et al. (1991)	Measures the frequency with which one engages in body image-related avoidance behaviors.

Mirror Focus Procedure	Butters and Cash (1987); Keeton, Cash, & Brown (1990)	Individuals look at themselves in a three-way mirror and then rate their personal level of discomfort.
Physical Appearance Behavioral Avoidance Test	Thompson et al. (1994)	Individuals approach their own image in a mirror from a distance of 20 feet; SUDS ratings and approach distance are dependent measures.
Cognitive measures		
Appearance Schemas Inventory	Cash & Labarge (1996)	Fourteen-item scale assesses core beliefs about appearance in females; three subscales (Vulnerability, Self-Investment, and Appearance Stereotyping).
Appearance Schemas Inventory—Revised	Cash, Melnyk, et al. (2004)	Twenty-item scale assesses beliefs and assumptions about the importance and influence of appearance in one's life on a 5-point Likert scale; has two subscales (Self-Evaluative Salience [12 items] and Motivational Salience [8 items]) and can be used with males and females.
Beliefs about Appearance Scale	Spangler & Stice (2001)	Twenty-item scale that measures beliefs about the consequences of appearance for relationships, achievement, self-view, and feelings on a 5-point Likert scale.
Body Image Automatic Thoughts Questionnaire	Cash et al. (1987)	Measures frequency with which females experience 37 negative and 15 positive body image cognitions.
Body Image Ideals Questionnaire	Cash & Szymanski (1995)	Ratings of personal ideal and actual rating on 10 attributes related to weight and appearance, along with the strength and importance of attribute.

(continued)

TABLE 10.1. *(continued)*

Name of instrument	Authors (year)	Description
Cognitive measures *(continued)*		
Body Image Ideals Questionnaire—Expanded	Szymanski and Cash (1995)	Ratings of the subject's specific attributes from a personal viewpoint and that of romantic partner based on "ideal" and "actual."
Body Weight and Shape Self-Schema	Stein & Hedger (1997)	Two 5-item scales that measure current and possible weight-related self-schema.
Bulimia Cognitive Distortions Scale—Physical Appearance Subscale	Schulman et al. (1986)	Measures degree of agreement with 25 statements that address physical appearance-related cognitions.
Drive for Muscularity Attitudes Questionnaire	Morrison et al. (2004)	Eight-item scale measures attitudes related to muscularity in males.
Modified Distressing Thoughts Questionnaire	Clark, Feldman, & Channon (1989)	Twenty-four-item scale containing anxiety-, depression-, and weight-related thought statements; individuals rate each statement for frequency and emotional intensity.
Physical Appearance Discrepancy Questionnaire	Altabe & Thompson (1995)	Based on Higgins's self-discrepancies questionnaire; indicate the physical appearance traits associated with one's actual, ideal, and cultural ideal self.
Swansea Muscularity Attitudes Questionnaire	Edwards and Launder (2000)	Twenty-item measure contains two subscales related to a muscular body image, drive for muscularity, and positive attitudes toward muscularity in males.

Perceptual measures		
Adjustable Light Beam	Thompson & Spana (1988)	Adjust width of four light beams projected on a wall to match perceived size of cheeks, waist, hips, and thighs of adult women.
Body Image Detection Device	Ruff & Barrios (1986)	Adjust width of light beam projected on a wall to match perceived size of a specific body site of adult women.
Digital Photography Mirror-Based Technique	Shafran & Fairburn (2002); Farrell et al. (2003)	Assesses whole body size estimation in adult females in an ecologically valid manner by means of their reflection in a full-length mirror, manipulating the image with digital photography to match perceived size.
Distorting Television Method	Bowden, Touyz, Rodriguez, Hennsley, & Beumont (1989)	Photograph distorted by video camera to 50% over and under actual size in adult women to assess perceived size.
Distorting Video Camera	Freeman et al. (1985)	Adjust a video image varied from 60% larger to 25% thinner in adult women to assess perceived size.
Image Marking Procedure	Askevold (1975)	Indicate perceived size by marking two endpoints on a life-size piece of paper.
Movable Caliper Technique: Visual Size Estimation	Slade & Russell (1973)	Adjust distance between two lights to match perceived size.
TV–Video Method	Gardner et al. (1987)	Adjust the horizontal dimensions of a TV image of oneself to match perceived size.
Video Distortion Method	Probst et al. (1998)	Adjust a life-size image projected onto a screen with a video camera to measure perceived size.

(continued)

TABLE 10.1. *(continued)*

Name of instrument	Authors (year)	Description
Subjective measures		
Body Esteem Scale—Children	Mendelson & White (1985)	Measures degree of agreement with various statements about the subject's body in boys and girls.
Body Esteem Scale—Adolescents and Adults	Mendelson et al. (2001)	Twenty-three-item scale for use with adolescents and adults with three subscales: Appearance, Attribution, Weight.
Body Image Assessment	Williamson et al. (1989)	Select from nine female figures that range from underweight to overweight and are presented in a random order.
Body Image Assessment—Revised	Beebe, Holmbeck, & Grzeskiewicz (1999)	Select from nine female figures that range from underweight to overweight.
Body Image Coping Strategies Inventory	Cash, Santos, et al. (2004)	Twenty-nine-item 3-point Likert scale assesses how individuals cope with various situations that threaten or challenge their body image; has three subscales (Avoidance, Appearance Fixing, Positive–Rational Acceptance).
Body Image States Scale	Cash et al. (2002)	Six-item scale assesses state body image in adult women.
Body Parts Satisfaction Scale—Revised	Petrie et al. (2002)	Fourteen-item scale uses a 6-point Likert scale to measure degree of satisfaction with various body sites in adult men and women.
Body Rating Scales for Adolescent Females	Sherman et al. (1995)	Adapted the adult version of the Figure Rating Scale for use with adolescent girls.

Body Satisfaction Scale	Slade, Dewey, Newton, Brodie, & Kiemle (1990)	Assesses degree of satisfaction with 16 body parts (general, head, and body subscales) in adult women.
Body Shape Questionnaire	Cooper et al. (1987)	Thirty-four items measure adult men and women's concern with body shape and size.
Breast/Chest Rating Scale	Thompson & Tantleff (1992)	Five male and five female schematic figures, ranging from small to large upper torso.
Color-A-Person Dissatisfaction Test	Wooley & Roll (1991)	Uses five colors to indicate level of satisfaction with body sites by masking on a schematic figure for both men and women.
Contour Drawing Rating Scale	Thompson & Gray (1995)	Nine male and nine female schematic figures, ranging from underweight to overweight.
Drive for Muscularity Scale	McCreary & Sasse (2000)	Fifteen-item measure uses a 6-point Likert scale to assess attitudes and behaviors related to muscularity in males.
Eating Disorder Inventory–2—Body Dissatisfaction subscale	Garner (1991)	Nine items use a Likert scale to assess dissatisfaction with specific body parts.
Figure Rating Scale	Stunkard, Sorenson, & Schulsinger (1983)	Select from nine male or female figures that vary from underweight to overweight.
Goldfarb Fear of Fat Scale	Goldfarb, Dykens, & Gerrard (1985)	Ten statements that reflect overconcern with fatness and body size.

(continued)

TABLE 10.1. *(continued)*

Name of instrument	Authors (year)	Description
Subjective measures *(continued)*		
Muscle Appearance Satisfaction Scale	Mayville et al. (2002)	Nineteen-item self-report measure assesses excessive concern with muscularity in males; has five factors (bodybuilding dependence, muscle checking, substance use, injury, and muscle satisfaction).
Multidimensional Body–Self Relations Questionnaire—Appearance Evaluation subscale	Brown et al. (1990)	Seven-item scale that measures overall appearance satisfaction in males and females.
Muscle Dysmorphic Disorder Inventory	Hildebrandt et al. (2004)	Thirteen-item scale consists of three subscales (Desire for Size, Appearance Intolerance, Functional Impairment) in males; uses a 5-point Likert scale.
Self-Image Questionnaire for Young Adolescents—Body Image subscale	Peterson et al. (1984)	Eleven-item scale assesses positive feelings toward the body in 10- to 15-year-old boys and girls.
Somatomorphic Matrix	Gruber et al. (1999); Cafri & Thompson (2004, plus additional unpublished data)	Systematically assesses muscularity and body fat dimensions in men and women; available in computer and paper-and-pencil forms.
Interview procedures		
Eating Disorder Examination	Fairburn & Cooper (1993)	Two of the four scales relate to body image: Weight and Shape Concern.
Interview for Diagnosis of Eating Disorders–IV	Kutlesic et al. (1998)	Contains multiple items that index DSM criteria for AN, AN, binge eating disorder, and EDNOS.

Structured Interview for Anorexic and Bulimic Disorders—Body Image and Slimness Ideal subscale	Fichter et al. (1998)	Semistructured clinical interview consists of six subscales, including Body Image and Slimness, which consists of 18 items related to body image disturbance.
Sociocultural and interpersonal influence measures		
Feedback on Physical Appearance Scale	Tantleff-Dunn, Thompson, & Dunn, (1995)	Twenty-six-item scale uses a 5-point Likert scale to assess verbal and nonverbal appearance-related commentary in adults.
Ideal Body Internalization Scale—Revised	Stice, Shaw, & Nemeroff (1998)	Ten-item measure assessing agreement with socioculturally endorsed views of the ideal woman.
Perceived Sociocultural Pressure Scale	Stice, Ziemba, Margolis, & Flick (1996)	Eight-item scale measures perceived pressure from the media, friends, and family to have a thin body.
Physical Appearance Related Teasing Scale	Thompson et al. (1991)	Eighteen-item measure assesses history of teasing related to weight, size, and general appearance.
Perception of Teasing Scale	Thompson, Cattarin, Fowler, and Fisher (1995)	Twelve-item scale indexing frequency and emotional response to general weight teasing and competency teasing.
Sociocultural Attitudes Towards Appearance Scale–3	Thompson et al. (2004)	Thirty-item questionnaire measures multiple aspects of societal influence on appearance and consists of four distinct subscales: Pressures, Information, Internalization–General, Internalization–Athlete.
Sociocultural Internalization of Appearance Questionnaire—Adolescents	Keery et al. (2004)	Five-item scale measures thin-ideal internalization in adolescent girls.

view for Anorexia and Bulimic Disorders has a body image scale as one of its six factors (Fichter, Herpertz, Quadflieg, & Herpertz-Dahlmann, 1998). Finally, the Interview for Diagnosis of Eating Disorders–IV includes symptom ratings for BID, as well as the other DSM criteria for AN, BN, binge eating disorder, and EDNOS (Kutlesic, Williamson, Gleaves, Barbin, & Murphy-Eberenz, 1998). (See Netemeyer & Williamson, 2001, for a more detailed description of these interview strategies.)

Most of the measures contained in Table 10.1 are quite simple questionnaire scales with items scored using a Likert format. A second type of measurement procedure, somewhat specific to the body image field, consists of the use of schematic or figural scales that contain images of individuals who differ in terms of body size (e.g., Thompson & Gray, 1995; Williamson, Davis, Bennet, Goreczny, & Gleaves, 1989). These scales offer an advantage in that they are easily understood, brief, and quickly scored. The essential strategy is to ask the patient to pick his or her ideal figure and current size; the discrepancy between the two ratings is taken as a measure of body size dissatisfaction. This index correlates highly with questionnaire measures of dissatisfaction (Thompson et al., 1999).

The vast array of possible measures for selection offers a somewhat daunting task for the clinician or researcher interested in choosing one or two brief scales to include in an assessment package. Certainly, a variety of factors should play into that decision (see Thompson [2004b], for a fuller discussion of this issue). First, it is important to include a measure of BID that will assess the weight-related dimension of dissatisfaction. Perhaps the most widely used measure in this area is the Eating Disorder Inventory–II, Body Dissatisfaction subscale (Garner, 1991); however, as Table 10.1 reveals, other measures also capture this dimension. Second, it may also be useful to include a measure that ascertains a more global, abstract notion of appearance concern; the Appearance Evaluation subscale of the Multidimensional Body–Self Relations Questionnaire (Brown, Cash, & Mikulka, 1990) is perhaps the most widely used scale to tap into this component of BID. This scale specifically addresses body image evaluation, which (as noted earlier) is how DSM-IV-TR characterizes the body image dysfunction for BN.

The decision to choose a scale from a specific category should depend on the specific nature of the assessment and desires of the clinician. For instance, often the patient may have specific aspects of BID (body-focused anxiety, negative cognitions, behavioral avoidance of body image-related situations, etc.) that are revealed from interview. Follow-up with specific BID measures designed to corroborate self-report might be indicated. Additionally, if some aspect of the treatment dealt with anxiety or emotional components of the eating problem, then an index of affective BID might be indicated. The same logic would apply to the selection of a cognitive or behavioral measure. Certainly, if some form of specific body image treatment is part of the comprehensive eating disorder treatment plan (e.g., Cash & Hrabosky, 2004), then pre and post assessment with a range of BID measures is indicated. Additionally, a good default option is to consider the inclusion of a measure from the generic subjective satisfaction category for all cases.

An important decision to make in the selection of BID scales is whether a state or trait measure is indicated for the specific research or clinical issue. The great majority of measures are trait measures; however, a few state measures have been developed. Primarily, these measures are used in experimental studies designed to reveal specific factors (for example, exposure to media images) that produce an immediate effect on BID (Thompson, 2004b). However, these measures are also ideal for use in a clinical setting as a gauge of the immediate within-session improvement in BID. One such measure is the State subscale of the Physical Appearance State and Trait Anxiety Scale (Reed, Thompson, Brannick, & Sacco, 1991). We have also used visual analogue scales, which are 100 mm. lines with the extreme descriptors at either end of the scale for the dimension under investigation (i.e., no appearance dissatisfaction—extreme appearance dissatisfaction) (Thompson, 2004b). Cash, Fleming, and Alindogan (2002) have also developed the Body Image States Scale, which is a series of five items designed to evaluate immediate changes in BID.

Another issue is the selection of a scale designed to specifically evaluate body dysmorphic disorder (BDD), which is an extreme form of BID consisting of a disparagement of some aspect of appearance that may border on the delusional. Certainly, there is the chance that BDD may be comorbid with an eating disorder, with the site of disparagement most likely a weight-related aspect of appearance (e.g., thighs, waist). However, according to the DSM-IV-TR, an additional diagnosis of BDD is not warranted unless the site of dysmorphia is clearly non–weight-related (e.g., nose, hair, etc.). The most widely used measure of BDD is the Body Dysmorphic Disorder Examination (BDDE; Rosen, 1996), which has 34 items that index symptoms of BDD.

Selection of a measure should always be guided by a careful evaluation of the psychometric qualities of the instrument and the validation sample for the specific scale. For instance, scales developed on adult white females may not necessarily be appropriate for use with an African American adolescent sample (Thompson et al., 1999). Many of the scales shown in Table 10.1 have normative and psychometric data for a range of age, gender, and ethnicity (such as the EDI and MBSRQ). Additionally, some scales have been developed specifically for use with adolescent samples such as the Self-Image Questionnaire for Young Adolescents (Peterson, Schulenberg, Abramowitz, Offer, & Jarcho, 1984). It is always useful to contact the authors of the scale for additional psychometric and normative data.

Another important issue with regard to measurement selection is the decision of whether to include a measure of the perceptual component of body image. Table 10.1 contains several widely used indices (see also Stewart & Williamson, 2004). However, recent work using sophisticated methods such as signal detection analysis question whether a true perceptual disturbance in body image exists (e.g., Thompson & Gardner, 2002). Signal detection allows for the differentiation of a reporting "bias" from a perceptual "sensitivity"; the latter has been assumed for many years to underlie the body size overestimation (distortion) typically reported for individuals with an eating disorder (especially AN) when compared to control participants (see Thompson, 1990). However, recent studies have found that even individuals with AN show a bias but little sensitivity when signal detection methods are used, leading Smeets, Ingleby, Hoek, and Panhuysen (1999) to conclude that individuals with AN show "normal sensitivity but an increased bias toward seeing stimuli as thinner" (p. 473). Therefore, it is our opinion that the use of perceptual measures in a clinical context should be undertaken with caution because the interpretation of findings using a simple procedure without an appropriate methodology (e.g., signal detection) may yield inaccurate results and interpretations.

The selection of a measure for use with boys or men is especially problematic given that many of the extant measures do not assess dimensions that are germane to the body image concerns of males. For instance, in recent years it has become clear that a muscular rather than a thin body is the ideal aspired to by most males (Cafri, Strauss, & Thompson, 2002; McCreary & Sasse, 2000; Pope et al., 2000). Pope and colleagues have even identified a clinical disorder that corresponds to a pathological pursuit of a muscular ideal, once referred to as "reverse anorexia" but now known as "muscle dysmorphia" (Pope, Gruber, Choi, Olivardia, & Phillips, 1997). In muscle dysmorphia, characterized as a subtype of BDD, a person typically experiences cognitive symptoms that include extreme body dissatisfaction and obsessive thoughts of not being sufficiently muscular, as well as behavioral symptoms like substance abuse (e.g., anabolic steroids), strict attention to dieting, and compulsive weight lifting and mirror checking (Olivardia, 2001). Two scales are available that provide for a measurement of muscle dysmorphia.

The Muscle Appearance Satisfaction Scale (MASS; Mayville, Williamson, White, Netemeyer, & Drab, 2002) consists of 19 items rated on a 7-point Likert scale. The items can be separated into five subscales: bodybuilding dependence, appearance checking, substance use susceptibility, injury, and muscle satisfaction. The Muscle Dysmorphic Disorder Inventory (MDDI; Hildebrandt, Langenbucher, & Schlundt, 2004) consists of 13 items rated on a 5-point Likert scale. The items assess three distinct factors related to muscle dysmorphia symptoms: desire for size, appearance intolerance, and functional impairment.

Other, more generic scales for the assessment of BID have also been developed for use with males. The Swansea Muscularity Attitudes Questionnaire (SMAQ; Edwards & Launder, 2000) is a 20-item measure containing two subscales assessing attitudes related to a muscular body image, drive for muscularity, and positive attitudes toward muscularity. The Drive for Muscularity Scale (DMS; McCreary & Sasse, 2000) is a 15-item measure with a 6-point response format that assesses attitudes and behaviors related to a muscular appearance. The Drive for Muscularity Attitudes Questionnaire (DMAQ; Morrison, Morrison, Hopkins, & Rowan, 2004) is an 8-item measure that assesses attitudes related to a muscular appearance.

RECENT ADVANCES

Perhaps the most impressive advance in the assessment of BID in recent years consists of the Somatomorphic Matrix, a bidimensional computerized body image test that can assess satisfaction with respect to muscularity and body fat for both females and males (Gruber, Pope, Borowiecki, & Cohane, 1999). The test consists of 100 generic figural human images arranged in a 10 × 10 matrix, representing 10 degrees of adiposity and 10 degrees of muscularity. Similar to other silhouette measures, the difference between ratings of one's own body and ideal body is interpreted as an index of dissatisfaction. In support of the measure's construct validity is that the images used correspond to particular FFMIs (fat-free mass indexes) and body fat percentages (Gruber et al., 1999). One limitation of the SM is its low test–retest reliability (Cafri, Roehrig, & Thompson, 2004), which led us to develop a paper-and-pencil modification consisting of 32 figures transposed from the original measure onto a 2 foot × 3 foot poster board, strategically placed in a matrix in order for the measure to cover the same domain as the 100 figures found in the original somatomorphic matrix (Cafri & Thompson, 2004). To make this measure more practical in application, we further reduced the number of figures to 16 (but still covering the same domain) and placed the figures on an 11 inch × 17 inch sheet of paper (Cafri & Thompson, 2004). The item reliabilities for this adaptation are slightly higher than those reported earlier for the original version of the Somatomorphic Matrix.

A second recent trend in body image assessment work is the development of a variety of measures designed to index constructs that are closely related to body image or that might be considered risk factors for the development of BID (see Table 10.1). For instance, as noted earlier in this chapter in the section on theoretical background, a variety of sociocultural forces such as media influences and psychosocial pressures (e.g., teasing) have been associated with the onset and maintenance of BID. Utilization of these measures may be useful not only for understanding factors connected to an individual's BID but also for pinpointing variables that may be associated with disturbed eating patterns (Levine & Harrison, 2004; Thompson, van den Berg, Roehrig, Guarda, & Heinberg, 2004).

SUMMARY

A variety of scales are available for the assessment of multiple dimensions of body image disturbance. The selection of a specific measure should be undertaken carefully, with the guiding logic of choosing measures that will provide for a multidimensional assessment that will prove useful not only for diagnostic purposes but also for the ongoing evaluation of treatment progress. Evaluation of the effectiveness of eating disorder treatment programs involves the measurement of many outcome variables. We hope that this chapter has provided some guidelines for the inclusion of body image disturbance measures in this endeavor.

REFERENCES

Altabe, M. N., & Thompson, J. K. (1995). Body image disturbance: Advances in assessment and treatment. In L. Vandecreek, S. Knapp, & T. L. Jackson (Eds.), *Innovations in clinical practice: A source book* (pp. 89–110). Sarasota, FL: Professional Resource Press.

American Psychiatric Association. (2000). *Diagnostic and statistical manual of mental disorders* (4th ed., text rev.). Washington, DC: Author.

Askevold, R. (1975). Measuring body image: Preliminary report on a new method. *Psychotherapy and Psychosomatics, 26*, 71–76.

Beebe, D. W., Holmbeck, G. N., & Grzeskiewicz, C. (1999). Normative and psychometric data on the Body Image Assessment—Revised. *Journal of Personality Assessment, 73*(3), 374–394.

Birch, L. L. (1990). Development of food acceptance patterns. *Developmental Psychology, 26*, 515–519.

Bowden, P. K., Touyz, S. W., Rodriguez, P. J., Hennsley, R., & Beumont, P. J. V. (1989). Distorting patient or distorting instrument? Body shape disturbance in patients with anorexia nervosa and bulimia. *British Journal of Psychiatry, 155*, 196–201.

Brown, T. A., Cash, T. F., & Mikulka, P. J. (1990). Attitudinal body-image assessment: Factor analysis of the Body Self Relations Questionnaire. *Journal of Personality Assessment, 55*, 135–144.

Bruch, H. (1962). Perceptual and conceptual disturbances in anorexia nervosa. *Psychosomatic Medicine, 24*, 187–194.

Butters, J. W., & Cash, T. F. (1987). Cognitive-behavioral treatment of women's body-image dissatisfaction. *Journal of Consulting and Clinical Psychology, 55*, 889–897.

Cafri, G., & Thompson, J. K. (2004). Measuring male body image: A review of the current methodology. *Psychology of Men & Masculinity, 5*, 18–29.

Cafri, G., Roehrig, M., & Thompson, J. K. (2004). Reliability assessment of the somatomorphic matrix. *International Journal of Eating Disorders, 35*(4), 597–600.

Cafri, G., Strauss J., & Thompson, J. K. (2002). Male body image: Satisfaction and its relationship to well-being using the somatomorphic matrix. *International Journal of Men's Health, 1*, 215–231.

Cafri, G., Thompson, J. K., Ricciardelli, L., McCabe, M., Smolak, L., & Yesalis, C. (2005). Pursuit of the muscular ideal: Physical and psychological consequences and putative risk factors. *Clinical Psychology Review, 25*, 215–239.

Cash, T. F. (1994). Body image and weight changes in a multisite comprehensive very-low-calorie diet program. *Behavior Therapy, 25*, 239254.

Cash, T. F. (1994). The Situational Inventory of Body-Image Dysphoria: Contextual assessment of a negative body image. *Behavior Therapist, 17*, 133–134.

Cash, T. F. (2002a). Cognitive-behavioral perspectives on body image. In T. F. Cash & T. Pruzinsky (Eds.), *Body image: A handbook of theory, research, and clinical practice* (pp. 38–46). New York: Guilford Press

Cash, T. F. (2002b). The Situational Inventory of Body-Image Dysphoria: Psychometric evidence and development of a short form. *International Journal of Eating Disorders, 32*, 362–366.

Cash, T. F., & Deagle, E. A. (1997). The nature and extent of body-image disturbances in anorexia nervosa and bulimia nervosa: A meta-analysis. *International Journal of Eating Disorders, 22*, 107–125.

Cash, T. F., & Fleming, E. C. (2002). The impact of body image experiences: Development of the Body Image Quality of Life Inventory. *International Journal of Eating Disorders, 31*, 455–460.

Cash, T. F., & Hrabosky, J. I. (2004). Treatment of body image disturbance. In J. K. Thompson (Ed.), *Handbook of eating disorders and obesity* (pp. 515–541). Hoboken, NJ: Wiley.

Cash, T. F., & Labarge, A. S. (1996). Development of the Appearance Schemas Inventory: A new cognitive body image assessment. *Cognitive Therapy and Research, 20,* 37–50.

Cash, T. F., & Pruzinsky, T. (Eds.). (2002). *Body image: A handbook of theory, research, and clinical practice.* New York: Guilford Press.

Cash, T. F., & Szymanski, M. L. (1995). The development and validation of the Body-Image Ideals Questionnaire. *Journal of Personality Assessment, 64,* 466–477.

Cash, T. F., Fleming, E. C., & Alindogan, J. (2002). Beyond body image as a trait: The development and validation of the Body Image States Scale. *Eating Disorders: The Journal of Treatment and Prevention, 10,* 103–113

Cash, T. F., Lewis, R. J., & Keeton, P. (1987, March). *Development and validation of the Body-Image Automatic Thoughts Questionnaire: A measure of body-related cognitions.* Paper presented at the meeting of the Southeastern Psychological Association, Atlanta, GA.

Cash, T. F., Melnyk, S. E., & Hrabosky, J. I. (2004). The assessment of body image investment: An extensive revision of the Appearance Schemas Inventory. *International Journal of Eating Disorders, 35,* 305–316.

Cash, T. F., Santos, M., & Williams, E. (in press). Coping with body-image threats and challenges: Validation of the Body Image Coping Strategies Inventory. *Journal of Psychosomatic Research.*

Cattarin, J., & Thompson, J. K. (1994). A three-year longitudinal study of body image and eating disturbance in adolescent females. *Eating Disorders: The Journal of Prevention and Treatment, 2,* 114–125.

Clark, D. A., Feldman, J., & Channon, S. (1989). Dysfunctional thinking in anorexia and bulimia nervosa. *Cognitive Therapy and Research, 13,* 377–387.

Cooper, P. J., Taylor, M. J., Cooper, Z., & Fairburn, C. G. (1987). The development and validation of the Body Shape Questionnaire. *International Journal of Eating Disorders, 6,* 485–494.

Durkin, S. J., & Paxton, S. J. (2002). Predictors of vulnerability to reduced body image satisfaction and psychological well-being in response to exposure to idealized female media images in adolescent girls. *Journal of Psychosomatic Research, 53,* 995–1005.

Dworkin, S. H. (1988). Not in man's image: Lesbians and the cultural oppression of body image. *Women and Therapy, 8,* 27–39.

Edwards, S., & Launder, C. (2000). Investigating muscularity concerns in male body image: Development of the Swansea Muscularity Attitudes questionnaire. *International Journal of Eating Disorders, 28,* 120–124.

Fairburn, C. G., & Cooper, Z. (1993). The Eating Disorder Examination (12th ed.). In C. G. Fairburn & G. T. Wilson (Eds.), *Binge eating: Nature, assessment, and treatment* (pp. 317–360). New York: Guilford Press.

Fairburn, C. G., Peveler, R. C., Jones, R., Hope, R. A., & Doll, H. A. (1993). Predictors of 12-month outcome in bulimia nervosa and the influence of attitudes to shape and weight. *Journal of Consulting and Clinical Psychology, 61,* 696–698.

Fairburn, C. G., Welch, S. L., Doll, H. A., Davies, B. A., & O'Connor, M. E. (1997). Risk factors for bulimia nervosa: A community case-control study. *Archives of General Psychiatry, 54,* 509–517.

Farrell, C., Shafran, R., & Fairburn, C. G. (2003). Body size estimation: Testing a new mirror-based assessment method. *International Journal of Eating Disorders, 34,* 162–171.

Fichter, M. M., Herpertz, S., Quadflieg, N., & Herpertz-Dahlmann, B. (1998). Structured Interview for Anorexic and Bulimic Disorders for DSM-IV and ICD-10: Updated (3rd) revision. *International Journal of Eating Disorders, 24,* 227–249.

Foster, G. D., Wadden, T. A., & Vogt, R. A. (1997). Body image in obese women before, during and after weight loss treatment. *Health Psychology, 16,* 226229.

Freeman, R. F., Thomas, C. D., Solyom, L., & Hunter, M. A. (1985). A modified video camera for measuring body image distortion: Technical description and reliability. *Psychological Medicine, 14,* 411–416.

Gardner, R. M., Martinez, R., & Sandoval, Y. (1987). Obesity and body image: An evaluation of sensory and non-sensory components. *Psychological Medicine, 17,* 927–932.

Garner, D. M. (1991). *Eating Disorder Inventory–2: Professional manual.* Odessa, FL: Psychological Assessment Resources.

Gilbert, S., & Thompson, J. K. (1996). Feminist explanations of the development of eating disorders: Common themes, research findings, and methodological issues. *Clinical Psychology: Science and Practice, 3,* 183202.

Goldfarb, L. A., Dykens, E. M., & Gerrard, M. (1985). The Goldfarb Fear of Fat Scale. *Journal of Personality Assessment, 49,* 329–332.

Gruber, A. J., Pope, H. G., Borowiecki, J., & Cohane, G. (1999). The development of the somatomorphic matrix: A bi-axial instrument for measuring body image in men and women. In T. S. Olds, J. Dollman, & K. I. Norton (Eds.), *Kinanthropometry VI* (pp. 217–231). Sydney: International Society for the Advancement of Kinanthropometry.

Heinberg, L. J. (1996). Theories of body image disturbance: Perceptual, developmental and sociocultural factors. In J. K. Thompson (Ed.), *Body image, eating disorders, and obesity: An integrative guide for assessment and treatment* (pp. 27–47). Washington, DC: American Psychological Association.

Heinberg, L. J., & Guarda, A. S. (2002). Body image issues in obstetrics and gynecology. In T. F. Cash & T. Pruzinsky (Eds.), *Body image: A handbook of theory, research, and clinical practice* (pp. 351–360). New York: Guilford Press.

Heinberg, L. J., Guarda, A. S., & Haug, N. A. (2001, December). *Sociocultural attitudes predict partial hospitalization weight gain.* Poster presented at the annual meeting of the Eating Disorders Research Society. Albuquerque, NM.

Heinberg, L. J., Haythornthwaite, J. A., Rosofsky, W., McCarron, P., & Clarke, A. (2000). Body image and weight loss compliance in elderly African-American hypertensives. *American Journal of Health Behavior, 24,* 163–173.

Heinberg, L. J., & Thompson, J. K. (1992). Social comparison: Gender, target importance ratings, and relation to body image disturbance. *Journal of Social Behavior and Personality, 7,* 335–344.

Heinberg, L. J., Thompson, J. K., & Matzon, J. L. (2001). Body image dissatisfaction as a motivator for weight loss: Is some distress beneficial? In L. Smolak & R. Striegel-Moore (Eds.) *Eating disorders: New directions for research and practice* (pp. 215–232). Washington, DC: American Psychological Association.

Hildebrandt, T., Langenbucher, J., & Schlundt, D. G. (2004). Muscularity concerns among men: Development of attitudinal and perceptual measures. *Body Image, 1*, 169–181.

Johnson, W. G., & Torgrud, L. J. (1996). Assessment and treatment of binge eating disorder. In J. K. Thompson (Ed.), *Body image, eating disorders, and obesity: An integrative guide for assessment and treatment* (pp. 321–344). Washington, DC: American Psychological Association.

Keery, H., Shroff, H., Thompson, J. K., Wertheim, E., & Smolak, L. (2004). The Sociocultural Internalization of Appearance Questionnaire—Adolescents: Psychiatric analysis and normative data for three countries. *Eating and Weight Disorders: Studies on Anorexia, Bulimia and Obesity*, 9, 56–61.

Keery, H., van den Berg, P., & Thompson, J. K. (2004). An evaluation of the Tripartite Influence Model of body dissatisfaction and eating disturbance with adolescent girls. *Body Image: An International Journal of Research, 1*, 237–251.

Keery, H., Boutelle, K., van den Berg, P., & Thompson, J. K. (in press). Teasing and body image disturbance: The role of the family. *Journal of Adolescent Health*.

Kutlesic, V., Williamson, D. A., Gleaves, D. H., Barbin, J. M., & Murphy-Eberenz, K. P. (1998). The Interview for the Diagnosis of Eating Disorders–IV: Application to DSM-IV diagnostic criteria. *Psychological Assessment, 10*, 41–48.

Larkin, J., Rice, C., & Russell, V. (1996). Slipping through the cracks: Sexual harassment, eating problems, and the problem of embodiment. *Eating Disorders, 4*, 525.

Levine, M. P., & Harrison, K. (2004). Media's role in the perpetuation and prevention of negative body image and disordered eating. In J. K. Thompson (Ed.), *Handbook of eating disorders* (pp. 695–717). New York: Wiley.

Levine, M. P., Smolak, L., Moodey, A. F., Shuman, M. D., & Hessen, L. D. (1994). Normative developmental challenges and dieting and eating disturbances in middle school girls. *International Journal of Eating Disorders, 15*, 11–20.

Mayville, S. B., Williamson, D. A., White, M. A., Netemeyer, R., & Drab, D. L. (2002). Development of the muscle appearance satisfaction scale: A self-report measure for the assessment of muscle dysmorphia symptoms. *Assessment*, 9, 351–360.

McCreary, D. R., & Sasse, D. K. (2000). An exploration of the drive for muscularity in adolescent boys and girls. *Journal of American College Health*, 48, 297–304.

Mendelson, B. K., & White, D. R. (1985). Development of self-body-esteem in overweight youngsters. *Developmental Psychology, 21*, 90–96.

Mendelson, B. K., Mendelson, M. J., White, D. R. (2001). Body Esteem Scale for adolescents and adults. *Journal of Personality Assessment, 76*, 90–106.

Morrison, T. G., Morrison, M. A., Hopkins, C., & Rowan, E. T. (2004). Muscle mania: Development of a new scale examining the drive for muscularity in Canadian males. *Psychology of Men and Masculinity*, 5, 30–39.

Netemeyer, S. B., & Williamson, D. E. (2001). Assessment of eating disturbance in children and adolescents with eating disorders and obesity. In J. K. Thompson & L. Smolak (Eds.), *Body image, eating disorders, and obesity in youth: Assessment, prevention, and treatment*. Washington, DC: American Psychological Association.

Olivardia, R. (2001). Mirror, mirror on the wall, who's the largest of them all? The features and phenomenology of muscle dysmorphia. *Harvard Review of Psychiatry, 9*, 254–259.

Oliver, K. K., & Thelen, M. H. (1996). Children's perceptions of peer influence on eating concerns. *Behavior Therapy, 27*, 25–39.

Peterson, A. C., Schulenberg, J. E., Abramowitz, R. H., Offer, D., & Jarcho, H. D. (1984). The Self-Image Questionnaire for Young Adolescents (SIQYA): Reliability and validity scales. *Journal of Youth and Adolescence, 13*, 93–111.

Petrie, T. A., Tripp, M. M., & Harvey, P. (2002). Factorial and construct validity of the Body Parts Satisfaction Scale—Revised: An examination of minority and non-minority women. *Psychology of Women Quarterly, 26*, 213–221.

Pope, H. G., Gruber, A., Choi, P., Olivardia, R., & Phillips, K. (1997). An under-recognized form of body dysmorphic disorder. *Psychosomatics, 38*, 548–557.

Pope, H. G., Gruber, A., Magweth, B., Bureau, B., deCol, C., Jovent, R., & Hudson, J. I. (2000). Body image perception among men in three countries. *American Journal of Psychiatry, 157*, 1297–1301.

Probst, M., Vandereycken, W., Vanderlinden, J., & Van Coppenolle, H. (1998). The significance of body size estimation in eating disorder patients: Testing the video distortion method on a life-size screen. *International Journal of Eating Disorders, 24*, 167–174.

Reas, D. L., Whisenhunt, B. L., & Netemeyer, R. (2002). Development of the Body Checking Questionnaire: A self-report measure of body checking behaviors. *International Journal of Eating Disorders, 31*, 324–333.

Reed, D. L., Thompson, J. K., Brannick, M. T., & Sacco, W. P. (1991). Development and validation of the Physical Appearance State and Trait Anxiety Scale (PASTAS). *Journal of Anxiety Disorders, 5*, 323–332.

Rieves, L., & Cash, T. F. (1996). Social developmental factors and women's body image attitudes. *Journal of Social Behavior and Personality, 11*, 63–78.

Rosen, J. (1996). Body dysmorphic disorder: Assessment and treatment. In J. K. Thompson (Ed.), *Body image, eating disorders, and obesity: An integrative guide for assessment and treatment* (pp. 149–170). Washington, DC: American Psychological Association.

Rosen, J. C., Srebnik, D., Saltzberg, E., & Wendt, S. (1991). Development of a body image avoidance questionnaire. *Psychological Assessment, 3*, 32–37.

Roth, D., & Armstrong, J. (1993). Feelings of Fatness Questionnaire: A measure of the cross-situational variability of body experience. *International Journal of Eating Disorders, 14*, 349–358.

Ruff, G. A., & Barrios, B. A. (1986). Realistic assessment of body image. *Behavioral Assessment, 8*, 237–252.

Shafran, R., & Fairburn, C. G. (2002). A new ecologically valid method to assess body size estimation and body size dissatisfaction. *International Journal of Eating Disorders, 32*, 458–465.

Sherman, D. K., Iacono, W. G., & Donnelly, J. M. (1995). Development and validation of body rating scales for adolescent females. *International Journal of Eating Disorders, 18*, 327–333.

Slade, P. D., & Russell, G. F. M. (1973). Awareness of body dimensions in anorexia nervosa: Cross-sectional and longitudinal studies. *Psychological Medicine, 3*, 188–199.

Slade, P. D., Dewey, M. E., Newton, T., Brodie, D., & Kiemle, G. (1990). Development and preliminary validation of the Body Satisfaction Scale (BSS). *Psychology and Health*, *4*, 213–220.

Smeets, M. A. M., Ingleby, J. D., Hoek, H. W., & Panhuysen, G. E. M. (1999). Body size perception in anorexia nervosa: A signal detection approach. *Journal of Psychosomatic Research*, *46*, 465–477.

Smolak, L., Levine, M. P., & Gralen, S. (1993). The impact of puberty and dating on eating problems among middle school girls. *Journal of Youth and Adolescence*, *22*, 355–368.

Smolak, L., & Murnen, S. K. (2004). A feminist approach to eating disorders. In J. K. Thompson (Ed.), *Handbook of eating disorders and obesity* (pp. 590–605). Hoboken, NJ: Wiley.

Smolak, L., Murnen, S. K., & Thompson, J. K. (in press). Body image disturbance and steroid use in adolescent males. *Psychology of Men & Masculinity*.

Spangler, D. L., & Stice, E. (2001). Validation of the Beliefs about Appearance Scale. *Cognitive Therapy and Research*, *25*, 813–827.

Stewart, T. M., & Williamson, D. A. (2004). Assessment of body image disturbance. In J. K. Thompson (Ed.), *Handbook of eating disorders and obesity* (pp. 495–514). New York: Wiley.

Stice, E., & Agras, W. S. (1998). Predicting the onset and remission of bulimic behaviors during adolescence: A longitudinal grouping analysis. *Behavior Therapy*, *29*, 257–276.

Stice, E., & Hoffman, E. (2004). Prevention of eating disorders. In J. K. Thompson (Ed.), *Handbook of eating disorders and obesity* (pp. 33–57). New York: Wiley.

Stice, E., Mazotti, L. Krebs, M., & Martin, S. (1998). Predictors of adolescent dieting behaviors: A longitudinal study. *Psychology of Addictive Behaviors*, *12*, 195–205.

Stice, E., & Shaw, H. E. (2002). Role of body dissatisfaction in the onset and maintenance of eating pathology: A synthesis of research findings. *Journal of Psychosomatic Research*, *53*, 985–993.

Stice, E., Shaw, H., & Nemeroff, C. (1998). Dual pathway model of bulimia nervosa: Longitudinal support for dietary restraint and affect-regulation mechanisms. *Journal of Social and Clinical Psychology*, *17*, 129–149.

Stice, E., Trost, A., & Chase, A. (2003). Healthy weight control and dissonance-based eating disorder prevention programs: Results from a controlled trial. *International Journal of Eating Disorders*, *33*, 10–21.

Stice, E., Ziemba, C., Margolis, J., & Flick, P. (1996). The dual pathway model differentiates bulimics, subclinical bulimics, and controls: Testing the continuity hypothesis. *Behavior Therapy*, *27*, 531–549.

Striegel-Moore, R. H., & Kearney-Cooke, A. (1994). Exploring parents' attitudes and behaviors about their children's physical appearance. *International Journal of Eating Disorders*, *15*, 377–385.

Striegel-Moore, R. H., Wilfley, D. E., Caldwell, M. B., Needham, M. L., & Brownell, K. D. (1996). Weight-related attitudes and behaviors of women who diet to lose weight: A comparison of black dieters and white dieters. *Obesity Research*, *4*, 109–116.

Stunkard, A. J., Sorenson, T. I., & Schulsinger, F. (1983). Use of the Dutch Adoption Register for the study of obesity and thinness. In S. Kety, L. P. Rowland, R. L.

Sidman, & S. W. Matthysse (Eds.), *The genetics of neurological and psychiatric disorders* (pp. 115–120). New York: Raven Press.

Szekely, E. A. (1989). From eating disorders to women's situations: Extending the boundaries of psychological inquiry. *Counseling Psychology Quarterly, 2,* 167–184.

Szymanski, M. L., & Cash, T. F. (1995). Body-image disturbances and self-discrepancy theory: Expansion of the Body-Image Ideals Questionnaire. *Journal of Social and Clinical Psychology, 14,* 134–146.

Tantleff-Dunn, S., & Thompson, J. K. (1995). Romantic partners and body image disturbance: Further evidence for the role of perceived-actual disparities. *Sex Roles, 33,* 589–605.

Tantleff-Dunn, S., Thompson, J. K., & Dunn, M. E. (1995). The Feedback on Physical Appearance Scale (FOPAS): Questionnaire development and psychometric evaluation. *Eating Disorders: The Journal of Treatment and Prevention, 3,* 332–341.

Thompson, J. K. (1990). *Body image disturbance: Assessment and treatment.* Elmsford, NY: Pergamon Press.

Thompson, J. K. (2004a). *Handbook of eating disorders and obesity.* New York: Wiley.

Thompson, J. K. (2004b). The (mis)measurement of body image: Ten strategies to improve assessment for clinical and research purposes. *Body Image: An International Journal of Research, 1,* 7–14.

Thompson, J. K., Cattarin, J., Fowler, B., & Fisher, E. (1995). The Perception of Teasing Scale (POTS): A revision and extension of the Physical Appearance Related Teasing Scale (PARTS). *Journal of Personality Assessment, 65,* 146–157.

Thompson, J. K., Coovert, D. L., Richards, K. J., Johnson, S., & Cattarin, J. (1995). Development of body image, eating disturbance, and general psychological functioning in female adolescents: Covariance structure modeling and longitudinal investigations. *International Journal of Eating Disorders, 18,* 221–236.

Thompson, J. K., Fabian, L. J., Moulton, D., Dunn, M., & Altabe, M. N. (1991). Development and validation of the Physical Appearance Related Teasing Scale. *Journal of Personality Assessment, 56,* 513–521.

Thompson, J. K., & Gardner, R. M. (2002). Measuring perceptual body image among adolescents and adults. In T. F. Cash & T. Pruzinsky (Eds.), *Body image: A handbook of theory, research, and clinical practice* (pp. 135–141). New York: Guilford Press.

Thompson, J. K., & Heinberg, L. J. (1999). The media's influence on body image disturbance and eating disorders: We've reviled them, now can we rehabilitate them? *Journal of Social Issues, 55,* 339–353.

Thompson, J. K., Heinberg, L. J., Altabe, M. N., & Tantleff-Dunn, S. (1999). *Exacting beauty: Theory, assessment and treatment of body image disturbance.* Washington, DC: American Psychological Association.

Thompson, J. K., Heinberg, L. J., & Marshall, K. (1994). The Physical Appearance Behavior Avoidance Test (PABAT): Preliminary findings. *The Behavior Therapist, 17,* 9–10.

Thompson, J. K., & Spana, R. E. (1988). The adjustable light beam method for the assessment of size estimation accuracy: Description, psychometrics, and normative data. *International Journal of Eating Disorders, 7,* 521–526.

Thompson, J. K., & Stice, E. (2001). Thin-ideal internalization: Mounting evidence for a new risk factor for body-image disturbance and eating pathology. *Current Directions in Psychological Science, 10*, 181–183.

Thompson, J. K., & Tantleff, S. T. (1992). Female and male ratings of upper torso: Actual, ideal, and stereotypical conceptions. *Journal of Social Behavior and Personality, 7*, 345–354.

Thompson, J. K., van den Berg, P., Roehrig, M., Guarda, A. S., & Heinberg, L. J. (2004). The Sociocultural Attitudes Towards Appearance Questionnaire–3 (SATAQ-3): Development and validation. *International Journal of Eating Disorders, 35*, 293–304.

Thompson, M. A., & Gray, J. J. (1995). Development and validation of a new body-image assessment tool. *Journal of Personality Assessment, 64*, 258–269.

Tiggeman, M., & Pickering, A. S. (1996). Role of television in adolescent women's body dissatisfaction and drive for thinness. *International Journal of Eating Disorders, 20*, 199–203.

Tsai, G., Curbow, B., & Heinberg, L. J. (2003). Sociocultural and developmental influences on body dissatisfaction and disordered eating attitudes and behaviors of Asian women. *Journal of Nervous and Mental Disease, 191*, 309–318.

van den Berg, P., Thompson, J. K., Brandon, K., & Coovert, M. (2002). The tripartite model of body image and eating disturbance: A covariance structure modeling investigation. *Journal of Psychosomatic Research, 53*, 1007–1020.

Veron-Guidry, S., Williamson, D. A., & Netemeyer, R. G. (1997). Structural modeling analysis of body dysphoria and eating disorder symptoms in preadolescent girls. *Eating Disorders: The Journal of Treatment and Prevention, 5*, 15–27.

Wertheim, E. H., Paxton, S. J., & Blaney, S. (2004). Risk factors for the development of body image disturbance. In J. K. Thompson (Ed.), *Handbook of eating disorders and obesity* (pp. 463–494). New York: Wiley.

Williamson, D. A., Davis, C. J., Bennett, S. M., Goreczny, A. J., & Gleaves, D. H. (1989). Development of a simple procedure for assessing body image disturbances. *Behavioral Assessment, 11*, 433–446.

Wooley, O. W., & Roll, S. (1991). The Color-a-Person Body Dissatisfaction Test: Stability, internal consistency, validity, and factor structure. *Journal of Personality Assessment, 56*, 395–413.

CHAPTER 11

Ecological Momentary Assessment

Scott G. Engel
Stephen A. Wonderlich
Ross D. Crosby

Eating disorder research has relied heavily on data gathered with instruments such as the Structured Clinical Interview for DSM-IV Diagnoses (First, Spitzer, Gibbon, & Williams, 1995) and the Eating Disorder Examination (Cooper & Fairburn, 1987). The use of these instruments has provided much valuable information about people with eating disorders. However, information garnered from self-report instruments has increasingly come under fire, and this has led some researchers to seek other means of gathering data. This chapter reviews a relatively new and innovative means of collecting data called ecological momentary assessment (EMA; Stone & Shiffman, 1994).

SELF-REPORT DATA AND ECOLOGICAL MOMENTARY ASSESSMENT

Self-reports are the primary source of data in psychology and the social sciences (Schwarz, 1999). In fact, it is difficult to think of many content areas in psychology in which traditional self-report (i.e., retrospective self-report) is not the standard means through which data are collected. Similarly, the vast majority of research conducted in the area of eating disorders has relied heavily on traditional self-report as a means of gaining knowledge. Despite the popularity and commonality of the use of traditional self-report measures today, these measures have a number of limitations that shape the conclusions that can be drawn from research in the many content areas where self-report dominates.

Some of the limitations of self-report are worth mentioning. Traditional self-report measures typically require participants to report on behaviors, beliefs, or feelings that occurred hours, days, weeks, or even years prior to their responding. For obvious reasons, simply forgetting accurate information is a concern when the recall period is considerable. Aside from simple forgetting, a wide range of memory biases have been identified in the last several decades (for reviews, see Schwarz & Sudman, 1994; Stone & Shiffman, 1994). For example, the recall of attitudes or emotions is consistently influenced by current attitudes or emotions (Markus, 1986; Teasdale & Fogerty, 1979). When one is in a bad mood, it is easier to recall negative events than when one is in a good mood. Also, when participants are asked to recall information about their behavior or mood over a longer time period (e.g., several weeks or months), the most salient and most recent events at the time of recall will disproportionately influence ratings of behavior or mood from the period that is being recalled (Redelmeier & Kahneman, 1996). As Smyth et al. (2001) point out, these limitations (and many more) have led some researchers to collect data in research laboratories rather than relying on participants to report information retrospectively. However, laboratory findings are also limited in terms of generalizability to the outside world. An example of this limitation can be seen in the phenomenon of "white-coat hypertension" (Pickering & Friedman, 1991). Many individuals have higher blood pressure readings when in a laboratory than when blood pressure is assessed in a natural setting. Also, moods may be systematically influenced in participants who take part in laboratory studies (Smyth et al., 2001). For example, it is possible that negative affect and anxiety may be increased in most subjects who participate in a study that takes place in a laboratory. Finally, poor convergent validity has been found between the physiological processes identified in the laboratory environment and those identified in natural settings. This poor convergence has been found for a host of physiological processes (e.g., Dimsdale, 1984; Houtman & Bakker, 1987; van Eck, Nicolson, Berkhof, & Sulon, 1996).

ECOLOGICAL MOMENTARY ASSESSMENT

Researchers have made many efforts to circumvent the aforementioned limitations of traditional self-report and laboratory-based research. One method of dealing with many of these limitations is daily diary research or experience sampling (Csikszentmihalyi & Larson, 1987) or Ecological Momentary Assessment (EMA; Stone & Shiffman, 1994). For the purposes of this chapter, all three of these very similar methods will be referred to as EMA.

EMA is highly portable and allows for the assessment of behavior and psychological states in the natural environment. It also allows for multiple daily data recording opportunities for participants, reducing the memory biases associated with traditional self-report measures. EMA typically involves signaling participants several times per day over a period of days or weeks. Signaling is completed through the use of electronic devices such as pagers, programmable wristwatches, and palmtop computers (Stone & Shiffman, 1994). The major advantage of EMA is the way it allows participants to provide data in a natural environment with minimal retrospective recall. Researchers in a wide variety of areas have made use of EMA: personality traits and affect (Bolger, 1990), asthma (Smyth, Soefer, Hurewitz, & Stone, 1999), dieting (Carels, Douglass, Cacciapaglia, & O'Brien, 2004; Carels et al., 2001), psychosocial interactions and mood (Stader & Hokanson, 1998), and chronic pain (Stone, Broderick, Porter, & Kael, 1997), to name a few.

Wheeler and Reis (1991) have described three EMA assessment methods to collect data: interval-contingent recording, signal-contingent recording, and event-contingent recording. EMA protocols are optimized when more than one of these formats is used, given that each approach has different strengths and weaknesses. Interval-contingent recording occurs at a fixed time interval during the assessment period (typically every 24 hours) and is often fixed around a particular event (e.g., bedtime). Signal-contingent recording involves the participant's completing a recording when signaled by an electronic device. The specific time that participants are signaled is determined by the investigator and is typically chosen randomly or semirandomly. Finally, event-contingent recordings require a participant to complete a recording after a predetermined event has occurred. For example, recording following a behavior of interest (e.g., binge eating episode) or an event of interest (e.g., stressful relationship event) would be examples of event-contingent recording. Each of these recording formats has strengths and weaknesses (see Wheeler & Reis, 1991, and Smyth et al., 2001) and should be chosen carefully, ideally in combination to adequately assess the variables of interest.

As noted, EMA reduces retrospective recall bias while allowing for assessment in a natural setting. In addition, EMA allows for the delineation of temporal ordering of variables of interest, which greatly enhances empirical assessments of cause and effect. Furthermore, EMA allows for the integration of models of proximal causal factors with more distal causal factors. For example, EMA could be used to test the hypothesis that early child abuse is associated with high levels of negative affect or emotional lability, which in turn is associated with binge eating. Additionally, EMA can be used effectively to test models that integrate state and trait variables. For example, the question of whether or not certain personality traits (e.g., emotional lability) moderate the relationship between stressful events and momentary mood could be effectively tested in an EMA paradigm.

EATING DISORDERS RESEARCH AND ECOLOGICAL MOMENTARY ASSESSMENT

While EMA is a relatively new technique, particularly in the area of eating disorders, a number of studies implementing it have been published in the relatively recent past. One recurring theme in these studies is the goal of teasing apart the temporal ordering of the variables of interest. The vast majority of EMA articles in the current literature on eating disorders are longitudinal studies investigating variables that are thought to cause or relate to eating disorder behavior in a particular temporal order.

Negative Social Interactions Precede Eating Disorder Behavior

For some time, research has suggested that negative social interactions appear to be associated with bulimia nervosa (BN; e.g., Cox, 1988). However, teasing apart whether negative social interactions are a consequence of some aspect of BN or whether bulimic behavior is preceded or caused by negative social interactions is very difficult to address using many traditional research designs and methodologies. This issue is particularly difficult to address in a natural environment without introducing the problem of retrospective recall. However, this issue has been addressed by three recent studies implementing EMA.

Okon, Greene, and Smith (2003) reported on 20 female participants with BN using EMA methodology. Participants were signaled eight times per day. Participants were asked about family stressors and bulimic symptomatology. Results indicated that for females who perceived their family as having high levels of conflict, family stressors preceded and significantly predicted bulimic symptomatology. While this finding may not address the etiology of BN, it provides information about the possible maintaining factors of bulimic symptoms.

Similarly, Steiger, Guavin, Jabulpurwala, Sequim, and Stotland (1999) used EMA methodology to investigate the impact of social interactions in BN (n = 55), former BN (n = 18), and women without eating disorders (n = 31). The participants in this study completed an EMA rating following all social interactions of 10 minutes or more. In these ratings, participants recorded mood, tone of the social interaction, self-criticism, and disordered eating symptomatology. Steiger et al. found that BN and former BN participants reported greater levels of self-criticism following negative social interactions than the other women in the study reported, suggesting that social stress and associated self-criticism may be significant variables in eliciting bulimic symptoms.

Past research has suggested that positive interactions with parents may serve as protective factors. While past cross-sectional research has suggested that positive relations with parents are associated with fewer eating disorder symptoms (e.g., Calam, Waller, Slade, & Newton, 1990), these studies could not delineate the temporal ordering of these variables. Swarr and Richards (1996) found that positive relationships with parents precedes (in this case by 2 years) and predicts more positive eating attitudes. It appears that while negative social interactions may causally relate to disordered eating behaviors in the short term, positive relations with parents may be causally related to fewer eating disorder symptoms over a longer period of time and thus serve as a potential protective factor.

Mood and Disordered Eating Behavior

Another area of eating disorder research that has made use of EMA methodology is the investigation of the mood–eating disorder behavior link. The first research study to investigate this relationship using EMA was conducted in the early 1980s. In a study well ahead of its time, Johnson and Larson (1982) signaled bulimic (n = 15) and control (n = 24) participants seven times per day inquiring about mood, mood variability, social isolation, and food-related behaviors. They found that when measuring mood at the momentary level, BN participants reported lower positive mood and higher negative mood as well as greater variability in mood overall. Also, they found that negative mood states preceded both binge and purge behaviors and that following a binge–purge episode, participants reported considerable increases in negative mood. Not only did this study make several groundbreaking findings regarding the mood–behavior link in eating disorder research, but it also laid the groundwork for future EMA research.

Another study that explored the relationship between eating disorder behavior and mood was conducted by Wegner et al. (2002). In this study, the investigators examined the relationship between mood and binge eating. They had 27 participants with subclinical binge eating disorders complete seven ratings per day for two weeks. Participants reported greater negative affect on days when they binged than on days when they did not binge. Contrary to hypotheses, worse mood did not appear to precede binge episodes, nor did it appear that improved mood followed binge eating. Somewhat discrepant from these findings, Greeno, Wing, and Shiffman (2000) found that patients with binge eating disorder did in fact report greater negative affect in the time leading up to binge eating. Similarly, Le Grange, Gorin, Catley, and Stone (2001) found that increases in negative affect and decreases in positive affect preceded binge eating in both participants diagnosed with binge eating disorder and those who did not receive a binge eating disorder diagnosis. Consistent with these findings by Le Grange et al., Steiger, Guavin, et al. (1999) found that poorer than average mood and lower self-concept ratings preceded binge episodes in BN patients. Further, following binge episodes, BN participants reported still lower mood and self-concept.

A recent study to investigate the mood–behavior relationship in BN was conducted by Wonderlich et al. (2004). This study was the first of its kind to examine the mood–behavior relationship in BN participants with a sufficient sample size to make relatively firm conclusions about the temporal ordering of mood and bulimic behavior. In this study, 131 BN participants completed ratings of mood, behavior (eating and other behaviors), stress, and coping. Through the use of EMA techniques, Wonderlich and his colleagues were able to show that high levels of negative affect and low positive affect preceded bulimic behavior, but this pattern varied by personality type, a point discussed further later in this chapter.

Finally, two studies have investigated the role of momentary affect in anorexia nervosa (AN). However, both studies had very small sample sizes and conclusions based upon the research in this area must be considered tentative at best. Larson and Johnson (1981) used EMA to gather information about two participants with AN. They found that these participants spent considerable time alone and that they reported considerable negative affect. Engel et al. (2004) collected EMA data from 10 participants with AN, investigating the interplay between cognitive discrepancies, mood, stressful events, and AN-related eating behaviors and rituals. These researchers found that among anorexic individuals, variability in affect predicted dietary restriction and ritualistic behaviors (r = .35) and that stressful events predicted variability in affect (r = .34) and dietary restriction and rituals (r = .58).

Moderating Effects of Trait Variables on State Variables

In addition to providing insight into the temporal ordering of variables (e.g., mood–behavior relationships), EMA allows researchers to study the interplay of trait and state variables. Further, EMA allows researchers to investigate how the relationship between state variables may be moderated by trait variables. For example, Steiger, Lehoux, and Gauvin (1999) found that in female BN participants ($n = 51$), momentary urge to binge was related to dietary control. However, this relationship was moderated by the participants' level of the personality trait of impulsivity. For participants with high levels of impulsivity, this urge to binge–dietary control relationship was not present, but this was not true of low-impulsivity subjects. The findings of Steiger, Lehoux, and Gauvin (1999) suggest that traditional therapies that target dietary control may be effective for low and moderately impulsive BN patients, but are not as effective for BN patients who are highly impulsive.

Another interesting study investigating the moderating effects of trait variables on the relationship between state variables was conducted by Wonderlich et al. (2004). As mentioned earlier, this study concluded that BN participants reported increased negative mood and decreased positive mood preceding bulimic behavior. More specifically, however, Wonderlich and his colleagues found that this mood–behavior relationship was moderated by personality. Conducting a latent profile analysis on 131 BN participants' personality indices, Wonderlich and his colleagues replicated past research (e.g., Goldner, Srikameswaran, Schroeder, & Livesley, 1999) suggesting that BN participants formed three naturally occurring groups: restricted compulsive, stimulus seeking–hostile, and low personality pathology groups. These three groups of BN participants reported different links between mood and bulimic behavior. While the restricted compulsive group displayed significant associations between negative mood and bulimic behaviors, the other two groups did not. This finding suggests that the postulated causal link between negative affect and behavior in BN may exist only for a subset of those with BN.

POSSIBLE LIMITATIONS OF ECOLOGICAL MOMENTARY ASSESSMENT

Feasibility

One of the key issues of concern with any EMA research study is the question of whether participants will be willing and able to complete the tasks we are asking them to do. Consistently, researchers have found in a wide variety of populations that participants show good to excellent compliance rates with EMA protocols. Not only do they comply with EMA protocols, they report the completion of the EMA recordings to be "easy," "a positive experience," "not very disruptive," and "not very time consuming" (Engel et al., 2004).

One way to demonstrate the feasibility of EMA research is to show that a good deal of research has been successfully completed using this methodology. To evaluate this question, we performed a PsycINFO search for the following three terms: "ecological momentary," "experience sampling," and "daily diary." From 1970 to 1980, these search terms resulted in the identification of four articles. From 1980 to 1989, the PsycINFO search identified 55 articles. From 1990 to 1999, these search terms produced 233 articles. Finally, in only the last 4 years (2000–2004) 224 articles were identified using EMA-related terms. Not only was there a dramatic increase in the number of articles that used EMA techniques, the variety of research areas and participant populations reported was also remarkable. Recent EMA research has been conducted on patients with osteoarthritis (Focht, Gauvin, & Rejeski, 2004), insomnia (Levitt et al., 2004), psychosis (Husky, Grondin, & Swendsen, 2004), depression (Peeters, Nicholson, & Berkhof, 2003), tic and habit disorders (O'Connor, Brisebois, Brault, Robillard, & Loiselle, 2003), sickle cell disease (Dampier, Ely, Brodecki, & O'Neal, 2002), and smoking (Shiffman et al., 2002), as well as participants who are college students (Pychyl, Lee, Thibodeau, & Blunt, 2000), and the elderly (Bouisson & Swendsen, 2003). Clearly, the research community has found that EMA techniques are both valuable and feasible in a wide range of content areas and with very diverse populations.

Reactivity

One of the key issues associated with EMA is that of reactivity. Reactivity occurs whenever the process of measuring a variable affects scores on that variable (Whitley, 1995). While reactivity has been a key concern with EMA since the advent of the methodology, little is known about the extent to which participants exhibit reactivity when being assessed through EMA techniques. To further complicate the issue, different areas of research are likely to have different concerns regarding reactivity. Hufford, Shields, Shiffman, Paty, and Balabanis (2002) found that undergraduate problem drinkers exhibited a very small amount of reactivity from EMA assessments. However, behaviors related to alcohol consumption may have very different reactivity-related concerns than behaviors associated with disordered eating. It has been argued that because eating disorder-related behaviors are much less socially acceptable, reactivity may be more of a concern for eating disorder researchers than those who study behaviors with less social stigma. However, the findings of Stein and Corte (2003) suggest that this does not appear to be the case. Stein and Corte had 16 BN and AN participants report a number of eating disorder-related behaviors on palmtop computers for one month. They then compared the frequency of these behaviors across different time intervals. Differences in frequency of reporting would suggest reactivity to the EMA assessment technique. However, differences in frequency of behaviors reported was not found, regardless of the time intervals inspected. Stein and Corte concluded that core eating disorder behaviors do not appear to be reactive to EMA assessment techniques.

Fleeting Affective States

Another limitation of EMA that has not been articulated in the literature is the duration of the variables of interest in eating disorder research. In particular, the study of mood and eating disorder behavior may be limited by the fact that states associated with disordered eating behaviors (e.g., see Heatherton & Baumeister, 1991) have been suggested to possibly be very fleeting (Smyth et al., 2001). For example, EMA-based research has not found that binge–purge behaviors result in reductions of negative affect (either temporary or long term) as suggested by past research (McManus & Waller, 1995). There are at least two possible reasons why improved affect has not been found following eating disorder-related behaviors using EMA methodology. First, it is possible that negative affect may not change following eating disorder-related behaviors. While this explanation is possible, it appears to be antithetical to behavioral principles. A more plausible explanation is that the absence of a reduction in negative affect is due to the requirements of the assessment process in EMA (and other self-report measurement processes as well). If the reduction is very fleeting (e.g., seconds or minutes), traditional self-report and EMA measures may not be able to assess the affective state soon enough after the behavior to capture the mood shift. Also, if reductions in negative affect occur as a result of some sort of distracted or even semidissociated state (Heatherton & Baumeister, 1991), the act of completing the EMA recording may require the participant to become more cognizant and thus put an end to this state.

Complexity of Statistical Analyses

One often underappreciated and overlooked difficulty in working with EMA methodology is the sheer complexity of the data collected. EMA protocols typically assess individuals at multiple time points throughout the day for periods ranging from several days to several weeks. This process can produce an enormous volume of data. For example, our recent EMA study of BN (Wonderlich et al., 2004) involved 131 participants completing a minimum of seven assessments per day over a 2-week period. This produced more than 13,000 separate data records. In addition to the volume, the structure of EMA data is typically complex. Individuals complete assessments at unequal and irregular time intervals, often complete differing numbers of assessments across days, and may differ in terms of the total number of days on which assessments are completed.

Given the complex, unbalanced structure common in EMA data, many of the statistical techniques familiar to most researchers (e.g., correlations, ANOVA, repeated measures ANOVA) are not appropriate for these data (Schwartz & Stone, 1998; Smyth et al., 2001). Researchers may be tempted to aggregate data over multiple observations (e.g., calculating means across days or subjects, tallying the total number of events) to simplify analyses. This can be problematic, however, for several reasons. Aggregation techniques fail to take into account the variability of multiple observations, which in itself may be an important clinical variable. In addition, aggregation strategies may mask potentially important patterns of variation across the course of a day or across days of the week. Aggregation across days may also produce problems of unequal error variance (Schwartz & Stone, 1998) and substantially diminish statistical power (Smyth et al., 2001).

A number of relatively recent statistical advances have led to the development of analyses appropriate for mixed-model unbalanced data of the type typically encountered in EMA protocols. These models have been variously referred to as random regression models (Gibbons, Hedeker, Waternaux, & Davis, 1988; Gibbons et al., 1993), random effects models (Laird & Ware, 1982), hierarchical linear models (Raudenbush & Byrk, 2002), or multilevel models (Snijders & Bosker, 1999). These models assume that observations are organized hierarchically; lower-level units are nested within higher-level units. In some applications, the upper-level units refer to groups, while the lower-level units refer to individuals who are members of these groups, such as students within schools (Raudenbush & Byrk, 1986). In other applications, the upper-level units refer to individuals and the lower-level units refer to repeated observations. For example, Bolger, Davis, and Rafaeli (2003) collected daily diary stress and coping data over a period of several weeks.

Applied to EMA data collection, these multilevel models are ideal for characterizing and evaluating the potential sources of influence on contemporaneous ratings such as mood. In this scheme, individuals (Level 3) are assessed across multiple days (Level 2) and provide multiple ratings within each day (Level 1). A person's mood at a given point in time may be a function of other Level 1 influences (e.g., events) in temporal proximity to the assessment. In addition, mood ratings at a particular occasion may also be influenced by Level 2 factors that vary from day to day, such as the day of the week (e.g., weekend vs. weekday) or the anticipation of a particular stressor on a given day. Finally, mood ratings at a particular point in time may be influenced by certain intrapersonal factors (Level 3), such as temperament or severity of eating pathology. These multilevel models thus allow estimation of variability associated with each of the three levels.

Multilevel models offer several advantages over more traditional analytic approaches to longitudinal data analysis (e.g., repeated measures ANOVA, MANOVA). Unlike traditional analytic models for longitudinal data, these models are appropriate for unequal group sizes, missing data on the repeated measure, and the measurement of subjects at different time intervals. Multilevel models also allow the inclusion of both fixed and time-varying covariates, provide individual parameter estimates for each subject, and allow the use of various covariance structures to account for the covariation of repeated or clustered observations (Schwartz & Stone, 1998; Krull & MacKinnon, 2001). Common covariance structures that can be used to model serial dependency include stationary and heterogeneous autoregression (AR), autoregressive moving averages (ARMA), and compound symmetry (CS). Likewise, time can be modeled in a variety of ways including simple linear, power polynomials, and exponential functions. Finally, the dependent variable itself can take a variety of forms. Random regression logit models have been developed for binary outcome data (Stiratelli, Laird, & Ware, 1984), generalized probit models have been developed for ordered categorical data (Hedeker & Gibbons, 1994), and mixed-effects Poisson models for count data (Albert, 1992; Siddiqui & Hedeker, 1997).

A number of excellent software programs are currently available that provide the resources for analyzing multilevel models. These include HLM-5 (Raudenbush, Byrk, Cheong, & Congdon, 2001), SAS PROC MIXED (Littell, Milliken, Stroup, & Wolfinger, 1996), the package of "mixed up" software programs (MIXOR, MIXREG, MIXNO, and MIXPREG) provided by Don Hedeker and Robert Gibbons at the University of Illinois at Chicago (Hedeker & Gibbons, 1996a, 1996b; Hedeker, 2001; tigger.uic.edu/~hedeker/mix.html), and *Mplus* Version 3 (Muthén & Muthén, 2004).

FUTURE DIRECTIONS FOR ECOLOGICAL MOMENTARY ASSESSMENT OF EATING DISORDERS

While EMA-based assessment has become increasingly popular in eating disorder research, the literature is still relatively sparse and would benefit greatly from further naturalistic investigation with EMA. Ironically, one of the areas that may benefit the most from further EMA is the same eating disorder research area where Johnson and Larson began it in 1982. The relationship between mood and eating disorder behavior is still far from well understood and future EMA protocols may be better able to disentangle the interplay between mood and eating disorder behaviors, as well as other antecedents and consequences. Further, virtually any area of eating disorder research in which temporal ordering of multiple variables may play a role in the maintenance or cause of eating disorder behaviors may potentially benefit from EMA.

Zetocha and McCaul (2004) recently added an innovative development to an EMA protocol. In traditional EMA fashion, they used palmtop computers to collect data. However, rather than merely implementing the palmtop computer as a receiver of information, Zetocha and McCaul also used the palmtop computer to manipulate the perceived control of smoking in approximately half of their sample. The manipulation of perceived control was accomplished several times during the day by using the palmtop computer to inform experimental participants whether they could or could not smoke their next cigarette. Contrary to the researchers' hypothesis, results suggest that participants in the low-perceived-control condition actually reported feeling more in control of their smoking behavior than those in the nonexperimental group.

The methods of this study are of particular interest. To the best of our knowledge, Zetocha and McCaul's (2004) study was the first to use a palmtop computer to both record information (i.e., EMA) and manipulate a variable of interest. This methodology could be fruitful in eating disorder research. For example, Wonderlich, Peterson, Mitchell, and Crow (2000) have proposed a model of BN in which negative emotional states precede and predict binge–purge behavior in BN patients. While traditional EMA assessment of negative emotional states and binge–purge behavior could provide valuable information about the etiology of BN, this relationship could also be experimentally tested with a methodology similar to that of Zetocha and McCaul. Negative emotional states could be manipulated with the palmtop computer (i.e. the experimental group could receive a manipulation that decreased negative emotional states) and both mood and binge–purge behavior could be assessed through typical methods with the palmtop computer. This is just one example of a variable that could be manipulated and assessment that could be conducted using a palmtop computer in eating disorder research.

Finally, another potential application of EMA is in conjunction with treatment. One study to investigate the role that EMA technology may play in treatment was conducted by Le Grange, Gorin, Dymek, and Stone (2002). These researchers sought to investigate how self-monitoring with palmtop computers could improve outcomes for patients with binge eating disorder. They found that self-monitoring with palmtop computers did not improve cognitive-behavioral treatment of these patients. Another study that implemented palmtop technology in treatment was conducted by Norton, Wonderlich, Myers, Mitchell, and Crosby (2003), who propose an application of palmtop computers as a component of a new treatment for BN. While they allude to the fact that data can be collected that may be used for research purposes, they primarily propose an innovative means of treatment delivery with the palmtop technology. These studies implemented palmtop technology as a tool in the treatment of eating disorders. EMA can potentially be used in eating disorder treatment outcome studies for both intervention and assessment. Information gathered through EMA may provide valuable information to therapist and researcher alike.

PRACTICAL APPLICATIONS OF ECOLOGICAL MOMENTARY ASSESSMENT

EMA has provided valuable information to researchers who study eating disorders. Technological advances such as palmtop computers have greatly enhanced the convenience of collecting real-time data. However, treatment providers may be left wondering how the method may be useful to them. Because we know that binge eaters report different behavior regarding their eating when they are in an interview than they report when using an EMA format (Le Grange et al., 2001), treatment providers may wish to make use of this information and collect real-time data from patients using a palmtop computer. By doing this, practitioners may discuss specific instances of eating-disordered behavior and address the antecedents and consequences of these symptoms in therapy. Further, clinicians may even wish to assess these antecedents and consequences of eating-disordered behaviors. For example, a clinician may set up a palmtop computer to assess bingeing and purging behavior as well as pre and post eating-disordered behavior mood and social interactions. This information could then be retrieved by the clinician at the participant's next scheduled appointment and be discussed during the session.

SUMMARY

EMA has aided in our knowledge of a number of areas of eating disorder research, but the methodology is still relatively new and many potential fruitful avenues have not been explored. Some research using EMA techniques has echoed past self-report findings, some has contradicted past research, and some has not been previously possible without the use of EMA. Further eating disorder research is needed using this methodology to help avoid the problems associated with laboratory studies and to better explore variables that are temporally associated with each other in the maintenance or etiology of eating disorders.

REFERENCES

Albert, J. (1992). A Bayesian analysis of a Poisson random effects model for home run hitters. *American Statistician, 46*, 246–253.

Bolger, N. (1990). Coping as a personality process: A prospective study. *Journal of Personality and Social Psychology, 59*, 525–537.

Bolger, N., Davis, A., & Rafaeli, E. (2003). Diary methods: Capturing life as it is lived. *Annual Review of Psychology, 54*, 570–516.

Bouisson, J., & Swendsen, J. (2003). Routinization and emotional well-being: An experience sampling investigation in an elderly French sample. *Journals of Gerontology, 58B*, 280–282.

Calam, R., Waller, G., Slade, P. D., & Newton, T. (1990). Eating disorders and perceived relationships with parents. *International Journal of Eating Disorders, 9*, 479–485.

Carels, R. A., Douglass, O. M., Cacciapaglia, H. M., & O'Brien, W. H. (2004). An ecological momentary assessment of relapse crises in dieting. *Journal of Consulting and Clinical Psychology, 72*, 341–348.

Carels, R. A., Hoffman, J., Collins, A., Raber, A. C., Cacciapaglia, H., & O'Brien, W. H. (2001). Ecological momentary assessment of temptation and lapse in dieting. *Eating Behaviors, 2*, 307–321.

Cooper, Z., & Fairburn, C. G. (1987). The Eating Disorder Examination: A semi-structured interview for the assessment of the specific psychopathology of eating disorders. *International Journal of Eating Disorders, 6*, 1–8.

Cox, C. R. (1988). Risk factors in the development of bulimia. *Dissertation Abstracts International, 48*, 3073.

Csikszentmihalyi, M., & Larson, R. E. (1987). Validity and reliability of the experience sampling method. *Journal of Nervous and Mental Disease, 175*, 526–536.

Dampier, C., Ely, B., Brodecki, D., & O'Neal, P. (2002). Characteristics of pain managed at home in children and adolescents with sickle cell disease by using diary self-reports. *Journal of Pain, 3*, 461–470.

Dimsdale, J. E. (1984). Generalizing from laboratory studies to field studies of human stress physiology. *Psychosomatic Medicine, 46*, 463–469.

Engel, S. G., Wonderlich, S. A., Crosby, R. D., Wright, T. L., Mitchell, J. E., Crow, S. J., et al. (in press). A study of patients with anorexia nervosa using ecological momentary assessment. Manuscript under review at *International Journal of Eating Disorders*.

First, M. B., Spitzer, R., Gibbon, M., & Williams, J. B. W. (1995). *Structured Clinical Interview for DSM-IV Axis I Disorders. Patient Edition (SCID-I/P)*. New York: Biometrics.

Focht, B. C., Gauvin, L., & Rejeski, W. J. (2004). The contribution of daily experiences and acute exercise to fluctuations in daily feeling states among older, obese adults with knee osteoarthritis. *Journal of Behavioral Medicine, 27*, 101–121.

Gibbons, R. D., Hedeker, D., Elkin, I., Waternaux, C., Kraemer, H. C., Greenhouse, J. B., et al. (1993). Some conceptual and statistical issues in analysis of longitudinal psychiatric data. *Archives of General Psychiatry, 50*, 739–750.

Gibbons, R., Hedeker, D., Waternaux, C., & Davis, J. (1988). Random regression models: A comprehensive approach to the analysis of longitudinal psychiatric data. *Psychopharmacology Bulletin, 24*, 438–443.

Goldner, E. M., Srikameswaran, S., Schroeder, M. L., & Livesley, W. J. (1999). Dimensional assessment of personality pathology in patients with eating disorders. *Psychiatry Research, 85*, 151–159.

Greeno, C. G., Wing, R. R., & Shiffman, S. (2000). Binge antecedents in obese women with and without binge eating disorder. *Journal of Consulting and Clinical Psychology, 68*, 95–102.

Heatherton, T. F., & Baumeister, R. F. (1991). Binge eating as escape from self-awareness. *Psychological Bulletin, 110*, 86–108.

Hedeker, D. (2001). *MIXPREG: A computer program for mixed effects Poisson regression*. Chicago: University of Illinois at Chicago.

Hedeker, D., & Gibbons, R. D. (1994). A random effects ordinal regression model for multilevel analysis. *Biometrics, 50*, 933–944.

Hedeker, D., & Gibbons, R. D. (1996a). MIXOR: A computer program for mixed-effects ordinal regression analysis. *Computer Methods and Programs in Biomedicine, 49*, 157–176.

Hedeker, D., & Gibbons, R. D. (1996b). MIXREG: A computer program for mixed-effects regression analysis with autocorrelated errors. *Computer Methods and Programs in Biomedicine, 49*, 229–252.

Houtman, I. L., & Bakker, F. C. (1987). Stress in student teachers during real and simulated standardized lectures. *Journal of Human Stress, 13*, 180–187.

Hufford, M. R., Shields, A. L., Shiffman, S., Paty, J., & Balabanis, M. (2002). Reactivity to ecological momentary assessment: An example using undergraduate problem drinkers. *Psychology of Addictive Behaviors, 16*, 205–211.

Husky, M. M., Grondin, O. S., & Swendsen, J. D. (2004). The relation between social behavior and negative affect in psychosis-prone individuals: An experience sampling investigation. *European Psychiatry, 19*, 1–7.

Johnson, C., & Larson, R. (1982). Bulimia: An analysis of moods and behavior. *Psychosomatic Medicine, 44*, 341–351.

Krull, J. L., & MacKinnon, D. P. (2001). Multilevel modeling of individual and group level mediated effects. *Multivariate Behavioral Research, 36*, 249–277.

Laird, N. M., & Ware, J. H. (1982). Random effects models for longitudinal data. *Biometrics, 38*, 963–974.

Larson, R., & Johnson, C. (1981). Anorexia nervosa in the context of daily experience. *Journal of Youth and Adolescence, 10*, 455–471.

Le Grange, D., Gorin, A., Catley, D., & Stone, A. A. (2001). Does momentary assessment detect binge eating in overweight women that is denied at interview? *European Eating Disorders Review, 9*, 309–324.

Le Grange, D., Gorin, A., Dymek, M., & Stone, A. (2002). Does ecological momentary assessment improve cognitive behavioural therapy for binge eating disorder? A pilot study. *European Eating Disorders Review, 10*, 316–328.

Levitt, H., Wood, A., Moul, D. E., Hall, M., Germain, A., Kupfer, D. J., et al. (2004). Pilot study of subjective daytime alertness and mood in primary insomnia participants using ecological momentary assessment. *Behavioral Sleep Medicine, 2*, 113–131.

Littell, R. C., Milliken, G. A., Stroup, W. W., & Wolfinger, R. D. (1996). *SAS system for mixed models*. Cary, NC: SAS Institute.

Markus, G. B. (1986). Stability and change in political attitudes: Observe, recall, and "explain." *Political Behavior, 8*, 21–44.

McManus, F., & Waller, G. (1995). A functional analysis of binge-eating. *Clinical Psychology Review, 15*, 845–863.

Muthén, L. K., & Muthén, B. O. (2004). *Mplus User's Guide* (3rd ed.). Los Angeles: Muthén & Muthén.

Norton, M., Wonderlich, S. A., Myers, T., Mitchell, J. E., & Crosby, R. D. (2003). The use of palmtop computers in the treatment of bulimia nervosa. *European Eating Disorders Review, 11*, 231–242.

O'Connor, K., Brisebois, H., Brault, M., Robillard, S., & Loiselle, J. (2003). Behavioral activity associated with onset in chronic tic and habit disorder. *Behaviour Research and Therapy, 41*, 241–249.

Okon, D. M., Greene, A. L., & Smith, J. E. (2003). Family interactions predict intraindividual symptom variation for adolescents with bulimia. *International Journal of Eating Disorders, 34*, 450–457.

Peeters, F., Nicholson, N. A., & Berkhof, J. (2003). Cortisol responses to daily events in major depressive disorder. *Psychosomatic Medicine, 65,* 836–841.

Pickering, T. G., & Friedman, R. (1991). The white coat effect: A neglected role for behavioral factors in hypertension. In P. M. McCabe, N. Schneiderman, T. M. Field, & J. S. Skyler (Eds.), *Stress, coping, and disease* (pp. 35–49). Hillsdale, NJ: Erlbaum.

Pychyl, T. A., Lee, J. M., Thibodeau, R., & Blunt, A. (2000). Five days of emotion: An experience sampling study of undergraduate student procrastination. *Journal of Social Behavior & Personality, 15,* 239–254.

Raudenbush, S. W., & Byrk, A. S. (1986). A hierarchical model for studying school effects. *Sociology of Education, 59,* 1–17.

Raudenbush, S. W., & Byrk, A. S. (2002). *Hierarchical linear models: Applications and data analysis methods* (2nd ed.). Thousand Oaks, CA: Sage.

Raudenbush, S. R., Byrk, A. S., Cheong, Y. F., & Congdon, R. (2001). *HLM-5: Hierarchical linear and nonlinear modeling*. Lincolnwood, IL: Scientific Software International.

Redelmeier, D. A., & Kahneman, D. (1996). Patients' memories of painful medical treatments: Real-time and retrospective evaluations of two minimally invasive procedures. *Pain,* 66, 3–8.

Schwartz, J. E., & Stone, A. A. (1998). Strategies for analyzing ecological momentary assessment data. *Health Psychology, 17,* 6–16.

Schwarz, N. (1999). Self-reports: How the questions shape the answers. *American Psychologist, 54,* 93–105.

Schwarz, N., & Sudman, S. (1994). *Autobiographical memory and the validity of retrospective reports*. New York: Springer-Verlag.

Shiffman, S., Gwaltney, C. J., Balabanis, M. H., Kenneth, S., Paty, J. A., Kassel, J. D., et al. (2002). Immediate antecedents of cigarette smoking: An analysis from ecological momentary assessment. *Journal of Abnormal Psychology, 111,* 531–545.

Siddiqui, O., & Hedeker, D. (1997). *Poisson random-effects models for correlated count data with applications*. Technical Report. Chicago: University of Illinois at Chicago.

Smyth, J. M., Soefer, M. H., Hurewitz, A., & Stone, A. A. (1999). Daily psychosocial factors predict levels and diurnal cycles of asthma symptomatology and peak flow. *Journal of Behavioral Medicine, 22,* 179–193.

Smyth, J., Wonderlich, S., Crosby, R., Miltenberger, R., Mitchell, J., & Rorty, M. (2001). The use of ecological momentary assessment approaches in eating disorder research. *International Journal of Eating Disorders, 30,* 83–95.

Snijders, T. A., & Bosker, R. J. (1999). *Multilevel analysis: An introduction to basic and advanced multilevel modeling*. Thousand Oaks, CA: Sage.

Stader, S. R., & Hokanson, J. E. (1998). Psychosocial antecedents of depressive symptoms: An evaluation using daily experiences methodology. *Journal of Abnormal Psychology, 107,* 17–26.

Steiger, H., Guavin, L., Jabalpurwala, S., Sequim, J. R., & Stotland, S. (1999). Hypersensitivity to social interactions in bulimic syndromes: Relationship to binge eating. *Journal of Consulting and Clinical Psychology, 67,* 765–775.

Steiger, H., Lehoux, P. M., & Gauvin, L. (1999). Impulsivity, dietary control and the urge to binge in bulimic syndromes. *International Journal of Eating Disorders, 26,* 261–274.

Stein, K. F., & Corte, C. M. (2003). Ecological momentary assessment of eating-disordered behaviors. *International Journal of Eating Disorders, 34,* 349–360.

Stiratelli, R., Laird, N. M., & Ware, J. H. (1984). Random-effects models for serial observations with binary response. *Biometrics, 40,* 961–971.

Stone, A. A., & Shiffman, S. (1994). Ecological momentary assessment (EMA) in behavioral medicine. *Annals of Behavioral Medicine, 16,* 199–202.

Stone, A. A., Broderick, J. E., Porter, L. S., & Kaell, A. T. (1997). The experience of rheumatoid arthritis pain and fatigue: Examining momentary reports and correlates over one week. *Arthritis Care and Research, 10,* 185–193.

Swarr, A. E., & Richards, M. H. (1996). Longitudinal effects of adolescent girls' pubertal development, perceptions of pubertal timing, and parental relations on eating problems. *Developmental Psychology, 32,* 636–646.

Teasdale, J. D., & Fogerty, F. L. (1979). Differential effects of induced mood on retrieval of pleasant and unpleasant events from episodic memory. *Journal of Abnormal Psychology, 88,* 248–257.

van Eck, M. M., Nicolson, N. A., Berkhof, H., & Sulon, J. (1996). Individual differences in cortisol responses to a laboratory speech task and their relationship to responses to stressful daily events. *Biological Psychology, 43,* 69–83.

Wegner, K. E., Smyth, J. M., Crosby, R. D., Wittrock, D., Wonderlich, S. A., & Mitchell, J. E. (2002). An evaluation of the relationship between mood and binge eating in the natural environment using ecological momentary assessment. *International Journal of Eating Disorders, 32,* 352–361.

Wheeler, L., & Reis, H. T. (1991). Self-recording of everyday life events: Origins, types, and uses. *Journal of Personality, 59,* 339–354.

Whitley, B. E. (1995). *Principles of research in behavioral science.* Mountain View, CA: Mayfield.

Wonderlich, S. A., Crosby, R. D., Engel, S. G., Mitchell, J. E., Smyth, J., & Miltenberger, R. (2004). *Personality grouping in bulimia nervosa: Differences in clinical variables and ecological momentary assessment.* Manuscript submitted for publication.

Wonderlich, S. A., Peterson, C. B., Mitchell, J. E., & Crow, S. J. (2000). Integrative cognitive therapy for bulimic behavior. In K. J. Miller & J. S. Mizes (Eds.), *Comparative treatments for eating disorders* (pp. 258–282). New York: Springer.

Zetocha, K. J., & McCaul, K. (2004). *Self-control and motivation to quit smoking cigarettes.* Unpublished manuscript, North Dakota State University.

CHAPTER 12

Treatment Planning

James E. Mitchell

The process of treatment planning generally requires input from several individuals, and unfortunately it is often not practical to have all these individuals come together to discuss the case. However, in situations where this is possible, such an approach is most effective. Clinics that see large numbers of patients with eating disorders often profit by having an intake clinic whereby subjects are evaluated in a variety of ways over a period of a day—by a psychiatrist or psychologist, a dietician, a pediatrician, internist, or family practitioner, and occasionally by other staff as well. With appropriate planning, staff can see several patients who rotate among them over the course of the day and then can meet in a group session to discuss their findings and plan treatment.

An alternative is to have a single individual responsible for treatment planning obtain information from other sources with complementary training and roles. This coordinator might arrange to have the patient evaluated by a physician for a physical examination and laboratory work, by a dietician for nutritional needs, and so on, and then consolidate the various findings into a treatment plan. Given that many patients with eating disorders are only marginally motivated for care and some are actively attempting to avoid it, whenever the evaluation activities can be conducted over a short period of time there is a higher likelihood that the individual will be captured by the system, and a coherent treatment plan can be implemented quickly.

For the evaluation to progress effectively it is ideal to have some information available to the team prior to actually seeing the patient. This may include a psychiatric database the patient can be asked to complete prior to the clinic visit or immediately before seeing the clinicians. It also might involve data from other health care providers who have worked with the patient in the past, including prior hospital and outpatient records, the results of any physical assessments, and the results of any recent laboratory work. Also, many dieticians find it useful to have patients self-monitor their eating behavior for a period of time before the assessment. Providing patients with forms on which to do so when they initially make their appointment can facilitate the process. Again, the more information available at the time of the evaluation, the more likely the system will be able to be responsive to the needs of the patient.

Treatment algorithms for patients with anorexia nervosa (AN), bulimia nervosa (BN), and binge eating disorder (BED) are shown later in this chapter in Figures 12.1, 12.2, and 12.3. Some of these algorithm recommendations are well established and empirically based (e.g., cognitive-behavioral therapy [CBT] for BN) while others are a bit more speculative and less supported by data (e.g., specific outpatient treatments for adult AN).

When the team is meeting to discuss a patient's treatment, it is most useful to begin with a brief overview of each professional's findings, followed by a synthesis from the team leader, whoever that may be. It is then reasonable to progress to consideration of a series of questions that can guide treatment planning:

1. Is this an emergency? Is the patient medically unstable? Is the patient suicidal?
2. If there is no urgent problem, what is the best level of care for this patient? Is the patient clearly already an outpatient treatment failure and in a need of a higher level of treatment? Is an outpatient trial practical?
3. A close correlate to question 2 involves the patient's insight and motivation. Is this patient coming to the clinic with some motivation for change? Or is the impetus coming from the family, while the patient has very little motivation?
4. What is the nature of the eating disorder? What is the patient's diagnosis? The core symptoms? What are the particularly problematic elements of eating disorder psychopathology? How critical is the patient's current weight? For AN patients, how much weight have they lost? How much do they need to gain?

5. What is the social support network like? If the patient is an adolescent, what is the situation in the family? Should the family be involved in treatment? Is there someone at home who can assist in treatment (for example, if a manual-based approach to adolescent AN is to be employed)?
6. What are the other psychopathological problems? These would include a whole spectrum of possible diagnoses ranging from depression to a family history of psychopathology.
7. What is the patient's knowledge of nutritional issues and what form of nutritional counseling is indicated?
8. What further medical evaluation needs to be done? Are there other laboratory tests that need to be monitored or laboratory abnormalities that need to be corrected? Should this be done in the emergency room today or in a physician's office in the next week?
9. Is the patient a candidate for pharmacotherapy? This is a particularly important question when evaluating outpatients with BN who are frankly depressed.

SPECIFIC TREATMENT RECOMMENDATIONS

This section provides an overview of therapy recommendations for patients with various diagnoses. Two assumptions underlie this discussion: that empirically validated therapies are preferable when they are available, and that many patients will benefit from a combination of psychotherapy and pharmacotherapy. In clinical reality, many therapists do not know how to deliver validated therapies for patients with eating disorders, and some have a bias against such manual-based therapies, seeing them as inherently restrictive for both therapist and patient, formulistic and unempathic. As someone who started his professional life trained primarily in psychodynamic psychotherapy and then progressed to a research career and an increasing focus on empirically validated manual-based approaches, I think that these criticisms are not justified. Most well-trained therapists with whom I have worked initially express concern about the lack of flexibility of such approaches, but the majority find them empowering, providing the therapist with guidance and tools often lacking in the usual therapy situation. There may be a growing divide between those who favor manual-based therapies and those who do not, but I firmly fall in the former group, while acknowledging that therapists at times need to diverge from specific guidelines for specific situations. I encourage therapists who work with patients with eating disorders to learn more about such therapies, as experiences with them will lead to enhanced skill and efficacy.

Anorexia Nervosa

Despite the fact that AN is a disorder with substantial morbidity and mortality, the empirical treatment literature on this condition is surprisingly small (Steinhausen, 2003; Sullivan, 1995). There are a number of reasons for this, including the low prevalence of the disorder, the variability in presentation, and the fact that many patients have a multiplicity of problems and therefore require several simultaneous interventions, which makes controlling for all the treatment variables in treatment trials difficult. Also anorexic patients are simply quite difficult to treat (Agras et al., 2004).

Relative to psychotherapeutic interventions, the number of adequately controlled randomized outpatient trials is again surprisingly scant and the literature is to some extent still primitive. For example, adherence to therapies has usually not been measured, and many times the assessment of outcome has not captured many of the core psychopathological variables seen in patients with AN. Many studies have also used less than optimal diagnostic interviewing techniques (Agras et al., 2004).

Certain published findings are interesting to consider since they have identified therapeutic elements that have not proven adequate in treatment. For example, nutritional counseling alone appears to be an inadequate approach. Also, very brief treatments for AN appear to be insufficient. By contrast, for younger patients still living at home, family-based interventions do appear to be helpful. In particular an approach originally developed at the Maudsley Hospital in London appears to have favorable results in some published work (Le Grange, Eisler, Dare, & Russell, 1992; Russell, Szmucker, Dare, & Eisler, 1987; Eisler et al., 2000; Dare, Eisler, Russell, Treasure, & Dodge, 2001; Lock, Le Grange, Agras, & Dare, 2001). Thus far, family therapy appears to have less utility with adults, and CBT, which has been used widely in the treatment of both BN and binge eating disorder, also appears to have some degree of efficacy in adults with AN, although it is usually offered for a longer period of time and in somewhat different ways than it is for these other conditions.

Relative to pharmacotherapy, most of the therapeutic trials that have been undertaken have been negative, yet in most of these studies the pharmacotherapeutic regimen has been added to some other treatment, which makes it difficult to examine the efficacy of the drug proper. Older antipsychotics, such as pimozide and sulpiride, do not appear to increase the effectiveness of an inpatient treatment program (Vanderycken & Pierloot, 1982; Vandereycken, 1984). However, more recent anecdotal work using the atypical neuroleptics, particularly olanzapine, suggest that these drugs may be helpful in decreasing obsessionality, improving mood, and increasing rate of weight gain in patients with AN; although the results are far from conclusive, and large multicenter randomized trials are needed (Allison, Mentore, & Heo, 1999; Newman-Toker, 2000; Powers, Santana, & Bannon, 2002; Carver, Miller, Hagman, & Sigel, 2002; Hansen, 1999).

Relative to antidepressants, one trial indicated efficacy for the older tricyclic antidepressant amitriptyline when added to inpatient treatment, but given its side effects and toxicity this drug is no longer used in this population (Halmi, Eckert, Ladu, & Cohen, 1986). The use of selective serotonin reuptake inhibitors (SSRIs), such as fluoxetine, does not appear to be helpful in underweight patients (Attia, Haiman, Walsh, & Flater, 1998), but in a limited amount of data appear to be associated with decreased rates of relapse after weight gain when combined with outpatient psychotherapy (Kaye et al., 2001). Lithium appears not to benefit patients with AN and can be frankly dangerous in these patients given their problems with fluids and electrolyte imbalances. A number of new agents are on the horizon, including corticotrophin-releasing hormone antagonists, which should be studied in these patients but which await adequate clinical trials.

To date,the drugs that may have some utility, given a very limited database, include atypical neuroleptics in underweight patients early in the course of treatment, and SSRIs used in combination with other techniques for relapse prevention purposes after the period of acute weight gain. For adolescents, a specific form of family therapy appears to be the best alternative. For adult patients the focus is less clear but current evidence favors an individual psychotherapy approach, primarily using a CBT model. However, it is important to remember that in addition to drugs and psychotherapy critically important elements of treatment in patients of AN are careful medical assessment and follow-up, along with nutritional counseling, as indicated in Figure 12.1.

As also shown in Figure 12.1, both partial hospital programs and inpatient programs have a particular role in the treatment of low-weight patients with AN. When it is available and when patients are at least to some degree cooperative, partial hospital programs are more cost-effective. However, not uncommonly full inpatient stays are necessary, particularly for those who are medically unstable or have failed in outpatient and at times partial hospital treatment. The same basic elements

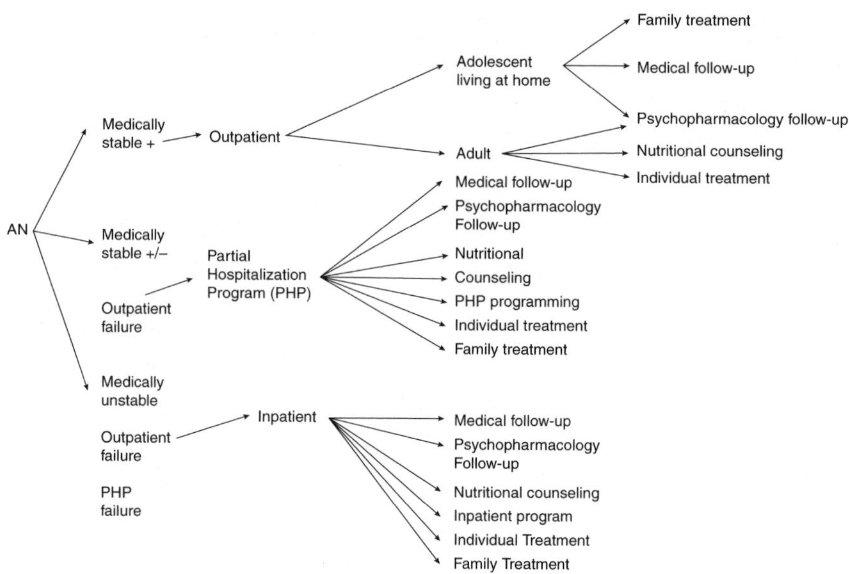

FIGURE 12.1. Treatment elements for anorexia nervosa.

need to be in place here, with more of an emphasis on supportive care and other programming including both group and individual therapy targeting the symptoms of anorexia.

Bulimia Nervosa

Of the available psychotherapeutic approaches that have been tested in empirical trials, CBT, whether administered in an individual or group format, appears to be the treatment of choice for BN, although interpersonal psychotherapy has also shown significant efficacy in two trials (Lee & Rush, 1986; Hay & Bacaltchuk, 2003; Fairburn, Jones, & Peveler, 1993; Agras, Walsh, & Wilson, 1999). The elements usually included in the CBT approach include self-monitoring, meal planning, an examination of cues and consequences, cognitive restructuring, and the use of relapse-prevention techniques.

Relative to pharmacotherapy a variety of antidepressants have been used in patients with BN and most appear to have some degree of efficacy (see, e.g., Walsh, Stewart, Roose, Gladis, & Glassman, 1985; Mitchell, Wonderlich, Peterson, & Crow, 2001; Hughes, Wells, Cunningham, & Ilstrup, 1987; Pope, Hudson, Jonas, & Yergelun-Todd, 1983). Fluoxetine is the only FDA-approved pharmacotherapy regimen for BN, and appears to be most effective when used aggressively at higher doses, such as 60 mg/day (Goldstein, Wilson, Thompson, Potuin, & Rampey, 1995; Fluoxetine Bulimia Nervosa Collaborative Study Group, 1992). The evidence from one large multicenter trial of fluoxetine suggests that the drug may be helpful in preventing relapse in patients with BN (Romano, Halmi, Koke, & Lee, 2002). There are also data suggesting that patients who do not respond adequately to CBT therapy may respond to antidepressant treatment with fluoxetine (Walsh et al., 2000).

Relative to the comparative efficacy of pharmacotherapy and psychotherapy, the results to date have been somewhat mixed (Agras, Rossiter, & Arnow, 1992; Mitchell, Pyle, et al., 1990; Bacaltchuk, Hay, & Trefiglio, 2003). In the best-designed trial reported to date, the advantage of adding antidepressant treatment to CBT alone was marginal (Walsh, Stewart, et al., 1997). However, many experts now would currently recommend adding pharmacotherapy to CBT in either of these cases:

- The patient is quite depressed at baseline (Mitchell, Peterson, Myers, & Wonderlich, 2001).
- The patient fails to evidence an early reduction in binge eating and purging frequency in CBT (e.g., less than 70% decrease by visit 7; Agras et al., 2000).

There also are studies showing that the 5-HT_3 antagonist ondansetron will suppress bulimic symptoms in a subgroup of patients, and that the anticonvulsant topiramate may have some antibulimic effects as well (Hartman, Faris, & Kim, 1997). Other treatments that have been studied but are currently not recommended include *d*-fenfluramine (which is no longer on the market), lithium, phenytoin, and naltrexone (Wermuth, Davis, & Hollister, 1977; Mitchell et al., 1989; Hsu, Clement, Santhouse, & Ju, 1991).

As shown in Figure 12.2, recommended outpatient treatments include CBT potentially combined with pharmacotherapy for adult patients. Much less is known about the treatment of adolescent patients with BN, although CBT and other therapies are beginning to be studied. Again the efficacy of pharmacotherapy in this age group is unclear. The question then becomes what to do with outpatient failures that have been treated with CBT and an adequate course of pharmacotherapy. The choice here is unclear, and in one trial the use of interpersonal therapy did not significantly improve outcomes after patients were treated with CBT (Mitchell et al., 2002). Some experts at this point would recom-

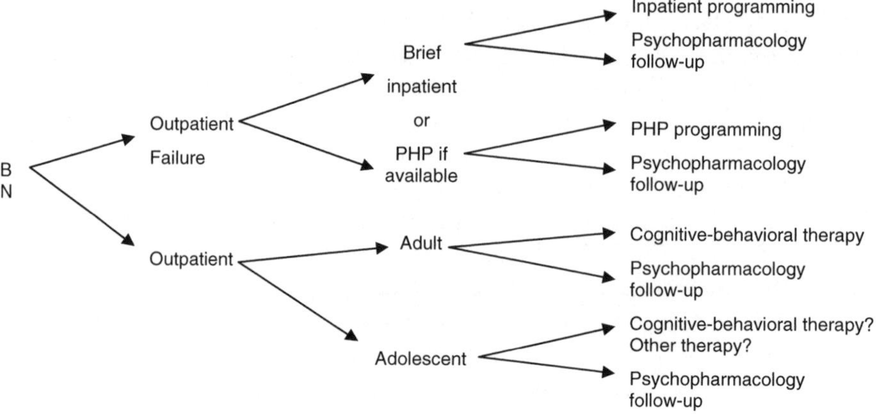

FIGURE 12.2. Treatment elements for bulimia nervosa.

mend a very brief inpatient or partial hospital stay to allow patients to gain control of their eating behavior, before reinitiating outpatient treatment.

Binge Eating Disorder

The treatment of BED remains controversial. This is attributable to the fact that when treating such patients, several potential targets are usually of concern, including (1) binge eating behavior, (2) overweight or obesity, and (3) comorbid psychopathology, particularly depression.

The current literature suggests that a variety of psychological and dietary treatments are at least moderately effective in treating BED resulting in significant improvement in binge eating at the end of treatment, and in some studies at long-term follow-up as well. However, weight loss has generally been limited in these trials.

Relative to specific forms of psychotherapy, similar to what has been shown in BN, structured forms of psychotherapy (such as CBT) that include many of the same elements have been shown to be quite effective in the treatment of patients with (Wonderlich, de Zwaan, Mitchell, Peterson, & Crow, 2003). Whether the addition of antidepressant medication improves outcome in these patients is unclear, with conflicting results to date (Grilo, Masheb, Heninger, & Wilson, 2002). Some evidence indicates that dialectic behavior therapy, a treatment originally developed for those with borderline personality disorder, can also be useful for patients with (Telch, Agras, & Linehan, 2001).

Relative to pharmacotherapy, the best established drugs thus far remain the antidepressants; a variety have been used, including most recently fluoxetine (Arnold et al., 2002), citalopram (McElroy, Hudson, et al., 2003), fluvoxamine (Hudson, McElroy, & Raymond, 1998), and venlafaxine (Malhotra, King, Welge, Brusman-Lovins, & McElroy, 2002). In most of these trials, patients experience a marked reduction in binge eating and modest, albeit perhaps clinically important, weight loss.

Relative to appetite suppressants, a large, well-controlled randomized trial of sibutramine indicated patients improved in terms of binge eating frequency and had a significant reduction in weight on active drug compared to placebo (Appolinario et al., 2003). A large multicenter trial of this drug has also been completed but the results are not yet available.

Relative to other agents, one trial demonstrated that topiramate, a drug originally introduced for the treatment of epilepsy, is useful in suppressing binge eating and causing significant weight loss (McElroy, Arnold, et al., 2003). The amount of weight loss with this drug has been particularly impressive and suggests that additional work needs to be done with it. In addition, an open-label trial of the anticonvulsant zonisamide appears promising (McElroy, Kotwal, Hudson, Nelson, & Keck, 2004).

Current recommendations for the treatment of BED are summarized in Figure 12.3. Patients need to be evaluated for their obesity in terms of their BMI and as to the presence of comorbidities such as dyslipidemias, hypertension, and Type II diabetes. These comorbidities will require additional treatment. Based on the degree of obesity, consideration should be given to various other types of interventions, including behavioral therapy and exercise combined with dietary modification in patients who are overweight, progressing through the use of pharmacological agents such as Orlistat and Meridia in patients who have a BMI greater than 30 or who are overweight and have significant comorbidities, and going as far as the

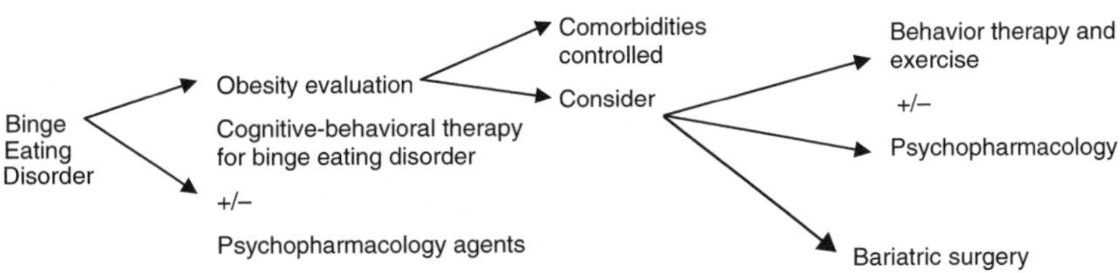

FIGURE 12.3. Treatment elements for binge eating disorder.

consideration of bariatric surgery in patients with a BMI greater than 40 or who have a BMI greater than 35 and comorbidities. Relative to the binge eating component, the treatment of choice at this time appears to be CBT, perhaps combined with psychopharmacological agents. However, the treatment algorithms for this condition are only now being developed and cannot be stipulated precisely at this time.

SUMMARY

A thorough review of the treatment literature on eating disorders is beyond the scope of this chapter. Instead, schematically, I have outlined general treatment guidelines for these illnesses. The clinician must address several issues simultaneously: necessary level of care, type of treatment, and choice of specific therapy. At this point in the development of treatments of eating disorders it is fair to conclude that our treatments for AN are not well established, but that the literature in this area is growing. The treatment for BN is better studied and more progress has been made here, but much is left to be accomplished, particularly for patients who fail to respond to CBT, antidepressants, or both. The treatment of BED is evolving, but a number of avenues are now being investigated. Clinicians who work with these patient groups need to continue to follow the literature as it moves forward.

REFERENCES

Agras, W. S., Brandt, H. A., Bulik, C. M., Dolan-Sewell, R., Fairburn, C. G., Halmi, K. A., et al. (2004). Report of the National Institutes of Health on Overcoming barriers to treatment research in anorexia nervosa. *International Journal of Eating Disorders, 35*, 549–555.

Agras, W. S., Crow, S. J., Halmi, K. A., Mitchell, J. E., Wilson, G. T., & Kraemer, H. C. (2000). Outcome predictors for the cognitive behavior treatment of bulimia nervosa: Data from a multisite study. *American Journal of Psychiatry, 157*, 1302–1308.

Agras, W. S., Rossiter, E. M., & Arnow, B. (1992). Pharmacological and cognitive behavioral treatment for bulimia nervosa: A controlled comparison. *American Journal of Psychiatry, 149*, 82–87.

Agras, W. S., Walsh, T., & Wilson, G. (1999, April). *A multi-site comparison of cognitive behavior therapy (CBT) and interpersonal therapy (IPT) in the treatment of bulimia nervosa*. Paper presented at the 4th International Conference on Eating Disorders, London, UK.

Allison, D. B., Mentore, J. L., & Heo, M. (1999). Antipsychotic-induced weight gain:

A comprehensive research synthesis. *American Journal of Psychiatry, 156*, 1686–1696.

Appolinario, J. C., Bacaltchuk, J., Sichieri, R., Claudino, A. M., Godoy-Matos, A., Morgan, C., et al. (2003). A randomized, double-blind, placebo-controlled study of sibutramine in the treatment of binge eating disorder. *Archives of General Psychiatry, 6*, 1109–1116.

Arnold, L. M., McElroy, S. L., Hudson, J. I., Welge, J. A., Bennett, A. J., & Keck, P. E. (2002). A placebo-controlled, randomized trial of fluoxetine in the treatment of binge-eating disorder. *Journal of Clinical Psychiatry, 63*, 28–30.

Attia, E., Haiman, C., Walsh, B. T., & Flater, S. R. (1998). Does fluoxetine augment the inpatient treatment of anorexia nervosa? *American Journal of Psychiatry, 155*, 548–551.

Bacaltchuk, J., Hay, P., & Trefiglio, R. (2003). Antidepressants versus psychological treatment and their combinations for bulimia nervosa. *Cochrane Database System Review, 4*: 2000.

Carver, A. E., Miller, S., Hagman, J., & Sigel, E. (2002, April). *The use of risperidone for the treatment of anorexia nervosa*. Paper presented at the Academy of Eating Disorder Annual Meeting, Boston, MA.

Dare, C., Eisler, I., Russell, G., Treasure, J., & Dodge, L. (2001). Psychological therapies for adults with anorexia nervosa: Randomized controlled trial of outpatient treatments. *British Journal of Psychiatry, 178*, 216–221.

Eisler, I., Dare, C., Hodes, M., Russell, G. F. M., Dodge, E., & le Grange, D. (2000). Family therapy for adolescent anorexia nervosa: The results of a controlled comparison of two family interventions. *Journal of Child Psychology and Psychiatry and Allied Disciplines, 41*, 727–736.

Fairburn, C. B., Jones, R., & Peveler, R. C. (1993). Psychotherapy and bulimia nervosa: Longer-term effects of interpersonal psychotherapy, behavior therapy, and cognitive-behavioral therapy. *Archives of General Psychiatry, 50*, 419–428.

Fluoxetine Bulimia Nervosa Collaborative Study Group. (1992). Fluoxetine in the treatment of bulimia nervosa. *Archives of General Psychiatry, 49*, 139–147.

Goldstein, D. J., Wilson, M. G., Thompson, V. L., Potuin, J. H., & Rampey, A. H. (1995). Long-term fluoxetine treatment of bulimia nervosa. Fluoxetine Bulimia Nervosa Research Group. *British Journal of Psychiatry, 166*, 660–666.

Grilo, C., Masheb, R. M., Heninger, G., & Wilson, G. T. (2002, November). A controlled study of cognitive-behavioral therapy and fluoxetine for binge eating disorder. Paper presented at the Eating Disorders Research Society Annual Meeting, Charleston, SC.

Halmi, K. A., Eckert, E., Ladu, T. J., & Cohen, J. (1986). Anorexia nervosa: Treatment efficacy of cyproheptadine and amitriptyline. *Archives of General Psychiatry, 43*, 177–181.

Hansen, L. (1999). Olanzapine in the treatment of anorexia nervosa. *British Journal of Psychiatry, 175*, 592.

Hartman, B. K., Faris, P. L., Kim, S. W., Raymond, N. C., Goodale, R. L., Miller, W. H., et al. (1997). Treatment of bulimia nervosa with ondansetron. *Archives of General Psychiatry, 54*, 969–970.

Hay, P. J., & Bacaltchuk, J. (2003). Psychotherapy for bulimia nervosa and binging. Cochrane Datatbase Syst Rev, 3, 2004.

Hsu, L. K., Clement, L., Santhouse, R., & Ju, E. S. (1991). Treatment of bulimia nervosa with lithium carbonate: A controlled study. *Journal of Nervous Mental Disorders, 179*, 351–355.

Hudson, J. I., McElroy, S. L., Raymond, N. C., Crow, S., Keck, P. E., Jr., Carter, W. P., et al. (1998). Fluvoxamine in the treatment of binge-eating disorder. *American Journal of Psychiatry, 155*, 1756–1762.

Hughes, P. K. Wells, L. A., Cunningham, C. J., & Ilstrup, D. M. (1987). Imipramine in the treatment of bulimia: A double-blind controlled study. *International Journal of Eating Disorders*, 6, 29–38.

Kaye, W. H., Nagata, T., Weltzin, T. E., Hsu, L. K., Sokol, M. S., McConaha, C., et al. (2001). Double-blind placebo-controlled administrations of fluoxetine in restricting- and restricting-purging type anorexia nervosa. *Biological Psychiatry, 49*(7), 644–652.

Le Grange, D., Eisler, I., Dare, C., & Russell, G. (1992). Evaluation of family treatments in adolescent anorexia nervosa: A pilot study. *International Journal of Eating Disorders*, 5, 599–615.

Lee, N. F., & Rush, A. J. (1986). Cognitive–behavioral group therapy for bulimia. *International Journal of Eating Disorders*, 5, 599–615.

Lock, J., le Grange, D., Agras, W. S., & Dare, C. (2001). *Treatment manual for anorexia nervosa: A family-based approach*. New York: Guilford Press.

Malhotra, S., King, K. H., Welge, J. A., Brusman-Lovins, L., & McElroy, S. L. (2002). Venlafaxine treatment of binge-eating disorder associated with obesity: A series of 35 patients. *Journal of Clinical Psychiatry, 63*, 802–806.

McElroy, S. L., Arnold, L. M., Shapira, N. A., Keck, P. E., Rosenthal, N. R., Karim, M. R., Kamin M., & Hudson, J. I. (2003). Topiramate in the treatment of binge eating disorder associated with obesity: A randomized, placebo-controlled trial. *American Journal of Psychiatry, 160*, 255–261.

McElroy, S. L., Hudson, J. I., Malhotra, S., Welge, J. A., Nelson, E. B., & Keck, P. E. (2003). Citalopram in the treatment of binge-eating disorder: A placebo-controlled trial. *Journal of Clinical Psychiatry, 64*, 807–813.

McElroy, S. L., Kotwal, R., Hudson, J. I., Nelson, E. B., & Keck, P. E. (2004). Zonisamide in the treatment of binge-eating disorder: An open-label, prospective trial. *Journal of Clinical Psychiatry, 65*, 50–56.

Mitchell, J. E. (2001). Psychopharmacology of eating disorders: Current knowledge and future direction. In R. Striegel-Moore & L. Smolak (Eds.), *Eating disorders: Innovative directions in research and practice* (pp. 197–212). New York: American Psychological Association Press.

Mitchell, J. E., Christenson, G., Jennings, J., Huber, M., Thomas, B., Pomeroy, C., et al. (1989). A placebo-controlled, double-blind crossover study of naltrexone hydrochloride in patients with normal weight bulimia. *Journal of Clinical Psychopharmacology*, 9, 94–97.

Mitchell, J. E., Halmi, K., Wilson, G. T., Agras, S., Kraemer, H., & Crow, S. (1999). A randomized secondary treatment study of women with bulimia nervosa who fail to respond to CBT. *International Journal of Eating Disorders, 32*, 271–281.

Mitchell, J. E., Peterson, C. B., Myers, T., & Wonderlich, S. A. (2001). Combining pharmacotherapy and psychotherapy in the treatment of patients with eating disorders. In A. E. Anderson (Ed.), *The Psychiatric Clinics of North America* (pp. 315–323). Philadelphia: Saunders.

Mitchell, J. E., Pyle, R. I., Eckert, E. D., Hatsukami, D., Pomeroy, C., & Zimmerman, R. (1990). A comparison study of antidepressants and structured intensive group psychotherapy in the treatment for bulimia nervosa. *Archives of General Psychiatry, 47*, 149–157.

Newman-Toker, J. (2000). Risperidone in anorexia nervosa: An atypical antipsychotic case study in AN. *Journal of American Academic Child and Adolescent Psychiatry, 39*, 941–942.

Pope, H. G., Jr., Hudson, J. I., Jonas, J. M., & Yurgelun-Todd, D. (1983). Bulimia treated with imipramine: A placebo-controlled, double-blind study. *American Journal of Psychiatry, 140*, 554–558.

Powers, P. S., Santana, C. A., & Bannon, Y. S. (2002). Olanzapine in the treatment of anorexia nervosa: An open label trial. *International Journal of Disorders, 32*, 146–154.

Romano, S. J., Halmi, K. A., Koke, S. C., & Lee, J. S. (2002). A placebo-controlled study of fluoxetine in continued treatment of bulimia nervosa after successful fluoxetine treatment. *American Journal of Psychiatry, 159*, 96–102.

Russell, G. F., Szmukler, G. I., Dare, C., & Eisler, I. (1987). An evaluation of family therapy in anorexia nervosa and bulimia nervosa. *Archives of General Psychiatry, 44*, 1047–1056.

Steinhausen, H. C. (2003). The outcome of anorexia nervosa in the 20th century. *American Journal of Psychiatry, 160*, 798. Sullivan, P. F. (1995). Mortality in anorexia nervosa. *American Journal of Psychiatry, 152*, 1073–1074.

Telch, C. F., Agras, W. S., & Linehan, M. M. (2001). Dialectical behavioral therapy for binge eating disorder. *Journal of Consulting Clinical Psychology, 69*, 1061–1065.

Vandereycken, W. (1984). Neuroleptics in the short-term treatment of anorexia nervosa: A double-blind placebo-controlled study with sulpiride. *British Journal of Psychiatry, 144*, 288–292.

Vandereycken, W., & Pierloot, R. (1982). Pimozide combined with behavior therapy in the short-term treatment of anorexia nervosa: A double-blind placebo-controlled cross-over study. *Acta Psychiatrica Scandinavica*, 66(6), 445–450.

Walsh, B. T., Agras, W. S., Devlin, M. J., Fairburn, C. G., Wilson, O. T., Kahn, C., et al. (2000). Fluoxetine for bulimia nervosa following poor response to psychotherapy. *American Journal of Psychiatry, 157*, 1332–1334.

Walsh, B. T., Stewart, J. W., Roose, S. P., Gladis, & Glassman. (1985) A double-blind trial of phenelzine in bulimia. *Journal of Psychiatric Research, 19*, 485–489.

Walsh, B. T., Wilson, G. T., Loeb, K. L., Devlin, M. J., Pike, K. M., Roosen, S. P., et al. (1997). Medication and psychotherapy in the treatment of bulimia nervosa. *American Journal of Psychiatry, 154*, 523–531.

Wermuth, B. M., Davis, K. L., & Hollister, L. E. (1977). Phenytoin treatment of the binge eating syndrome. *American Journal of Psychiatry, 134*, 1249–1253.

Wonderlich, S. A., de Zwaan, M., Mitchell, J. E., Peterson C., & Crow, S. (2003). Psychological and dietary treatment of binge eating disorder: Conceptual implications. *International Journal of Eating Disorders, 34*, S58-S73.

Index